Contemporary Mental Health: Theory, Policy and Practice

At the beginning of the twenty-first century, mental health services in England and Wales are at a critical point in terms of their development. This book considers a number of key themes and tensions in relation to theory, policy, practice and research, emphasizing the complex relationships between these four areas and exploring the impact of service user, carer and professional perspectives.

Contemporary Mental Health: Theory, Policy and Practice examines the tensions between different professional models, varying 'social' perspectives and political imperatives and explores how these tensions are manifested in practice. Topics covered include:

- the emphasis on risk as opposed to citizenship and entitlement;
- social exclusion and inclusion;
- professional and user perspectives;
- the 'territories' of health and social care and their respective roles and relationships.

An important theme running throughout is the critical appraisal of perspectives concerning gender, ethnicity and sexuality, drawing out wider issues of power and inequality.

Contemporary Mental Health: Theory, Policy and Practice makes ideas and theoretical policy material accessible and applicable, and is a key text for students and practitioners in mental health, social work and social care.

Barbara Fawcett is Professor of Social Work and Policy Studies at the University of Sydney. Previous appointments include Head of the Department of Social Sciences and Humanities at the University of Bradford. She has considerable experience in the field having worked as a psychiatric social worker, manager, senior manager and research consultant in the field of mental health.

Kate Karban is Principal Lecturer in Mental Health at Leeds Metropolitan University and has been involved in social work and mental health education and training. She has a background in mental health and social work in a variety of settings.

Contemporary Mental Health: Theory, Policy and Practice

Barbara Fawcett and Kate Karban

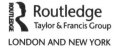
Routledge
Taylor & Francis Group

LONDON AND NEW YORK

First published in 2005 by Routledge
2 Park Square, Milton Park, Abingdon, Oxon OX14 4RN
Simultaneously published in the USA and Canada
by Routledge
270 Madison Avenue, New York, NY 10016

Routledge is an imprint of the Taylor and Francis Group

Transferred to Digital Printing 2006

Taylor and Francis Group is the Academic Division of TandF Informa plc

© 2005 Barbara Fawcett and Kate Karban

Typeset in 10/12 Sabon by Scribe Design Ltd, Ashford, UK

British Library Cataloguing in Publication Data

A catalogue record for this book is available from the British
Library

Library of Congress Cataloging in Publication Data
A catalogue record has been requested

ISBN 0 415 32845 4(hbk)
ISBN 0 415 32846 2(pbk)

Publisher's Note
The publisher has gone to great lengths to ensure the quality of this reprint
but points out that some imperfections in the original may be apparent

Contents

Dedication

Dedicated to Sophie and Katie and Laura and Alex

Acknowledgements

We would like to thank Maurice Hanlon and Brid Featherstone for reading drafts of this book.

1 Introduction

Madness! Madness!

(Closing line to *The Bridge on the River Kwai* 1957).

What is 'madness'? What is 'sanity'? These are questions that have preoccupied philosophers, physicians and more recently psychiatrists, psychologists and sociologists. In a similar vein, when we talk about these areas are we talking about health and by definition mental health and ill-health or something else? If we focus on mental well-being or health, when does mental ill-health become illness? How are the dividing lines between those regarded as mentally healthy or mentally ill drawn and what part do prevailing ideologies, social and cultural practices and belief systems play in understandings, definitions and identification processes? These are all questions that will be explored in this book as theoretical and historical underpinnings of current ways of thinking are examined, prevailing policy is appraised and the implications for practice and for those utilizing current service provision are reviewed.

As a major aim of the book is to enable the reader to navigate the complex terrain that is occupied by understandings of 'mental health', emphasis is placed on the route from theory to policy to practice and back again. In order to facilitate critical reflection, it is not the intention to provide a new model or paradigm, but to provide accessible links between practice and praxis which incorporates the identification of conceptual signposts. It is argued that it is not so much 'what' individuals understand and apply, but 'how' they make connections between theory, policy and practice and 'how' they make dynamic and flexible use of knowledge, skills, values, analysis and evaluative methodology, that ought to be the object of attention. As part of this flexible map, individuals are charged with both locating the ways in which they are positioning themselves and locating the ways in which they are positioned by the operation of prevailing power relationships and paradigms. The experience of all individuals including those who utilize as well as those who provide services is important here. This is not to interpret experience as something that can be applied in a universalistic and standardized way to all situations, but to view it as an attribute which needs to be reflexively applied in a situationally specific manner. It is also important that the paradox, tension and inconsistency which can be seen to be integrally contained within policy and practice are not glossed over, but emphasized to draw attention to difference and diversity and the variety of conceptual paradigms operating.

However, at the outset, it is important to look at the current terminology used, the implications of the various names and labels and why particular terms have been chosen for this book. Clearly any exploration of this area immediately raises ontological and epistemological questions about how the questioner understands 'madness' and 'sanity' and the ways in which knowledge frameworks are applied. Taking this on board, terms and phrases in current usage include mental health, mental ill-health, mental illness, severe psychological distress, mental distress, problems with living, and madness. Those perceived, or who perceive themselves, to be experiencing difficulties can use or have applied to them a range of terms with the most common being 'patient', 'ex-patient', 'client', 'service user', 'user', 'consumer' and 'survivor'. The terms used influence how an individual or group is viewed and how they view themselves. Labels and associated dichotomies, such as psychiatrist/patient, service provider/service user, easily become entrenched with expert opinion being regarded as the legitimate form of knowledge and forms of experience being ignored and marginalized. These distinctions similarly fail to highlight that 'mental ill-health' or 'mental distress', albeit in varying forms and to different degrees, is experienced by everyone. Some manage distress alone or informally with the assistance of family or friends, some choose or have chosen for them more formal support either privately or through publicly funded services. The form that this support takes can vary between professionally supervised drug treatments, talking therapies and alternative approaches such as becoming a member of the 'Hearing Voices' network, or a combination. There is also the issue of involuntary detention and/or treatment to consider. Some argue that this is never justified and that the criminal and civil laws that apply to everyone are all that is required (for example, Szasz 1971; Grobe 1995). Others maintain that the protection of the public and the self-protection of the individual diagnosed as having a 'mental disorder' have to be prioritized (for example, Howe 1995). Barnes and Bowl (2001) steer a course between these positions. They state: 'It is important to recognise that there *are* times when uninvited interventions may, in the long run, be capable of creating the conditions in which empowerment is possible and a failure to act on the part of mental health workers is the most destructive response' (2001: 4).

This overview draws attention not only to the difficulties associated with defining 'mental health' or 'mental distress' but also to the current overriding emphasis on medicalized understandings and practice responses. However, in this context, it is all too easy to set up a categorical distinction between 'medical' and 'social' orientations or Eurocentric and non-Eurocentric perspectives and to imply that there are rigid divisions, a lack of overlap, an absence of shared features, or that one should be prioritized over another. Rather than going down this particular path, this book is concerned with exploring the meanings associated with, to use the broad-brush term, mental distress,[1] utilizing critiques which draw from wide-ranging forms of analyses. Adherence to one perspective or one model is eschewed in favour of concentrating on the importance of the ongoing interrogation of situational factors, of broader-based understandings and the acknowledged and unacknowledged value judgements which inform action and practices. This is not to downplay the significance of mental ill-health/mental distress as such. Wilson and Beresford (2002) when discussing the socially constructed nature of mental illness assert: 'we do not wish to deny or play down the very real mental and emotional distress that we and other psychiatric system survivors experience. We nevertheless view this as part of a broader continuum of distress and well-being: a continuum upon which all people would place themselves, in different positions and at different times in their lives' (2002: 144). This is the view adopted in this book with regard to how both individual experience and constructing processes are both acknowledged and appraised.

The effects and consequences of increasing globalization and associated debates in relation to understandings of mental distress also require attention at this point. Discussion about the nature and consequences of globalization are wide-ranging. Initially driven by economic concerns and critiques directed at the cost of the welfare state, strongly regulated economies and high taxation systems, attention has increasingly turned to issues related to the standardization of policies and practices in a wide range of areas. However, Fook (2002) points out that one of the difficulties, but also one of the challenges, of understanding globalization is recognizing the ways in which world-scale changes have different and contradictory expressions in different contexts. With regard to the maintenance of cultural differences in the face of encroaching globalization, Kirmayer (2001) acknowledges that in relation to psychiatry, culture influences the sources, symptoms and idioms of distress, as well as individuals' explanatory models, coping mechanisms and help-seeking behaviour and their social responses to distress and disability. Bhungra and Mastrogianni (2004) contend that, despite the influence of mass media and electronic telecommunication, widespread homogenization with regard to cultural understandings of mental health is not taking place. This they attribute to the process of globalization affecting only a minority and being counteracted by the reassertion of ethnic identities. They regard an increase in urbanization with its related rootlessness as being associated with globalization, but see

---

1 Where appropriate the term 'mental health' has also been used.

this as having a wider-ranging significance with regard to the causative aspects of mental distress. These perspectives draw attention to the implications of globalization being far from straightforward and key aspects will be referred to throughout the book.

STRUCTURE OF THE BOOK

This book is divided into two main sections. The first, entitled 'Theory, policy and tensions', incorporates Chapters 2, 3, 4 and 5. These explore the theoretical underpinnings to current understandings in the arena of mental health and appraise the historical and contemporary policy framework. In this section issues of inclusiveness and exclusiveness are examined, with particular attention being paid to the influence of gender and ethnicity. The embedded tension, paradox and inconsistency apparent in the current policy framework are also subject to critical scrutiny. The second section, entitled 'The changing contemporary scene: forwards – backwards?', contains Chapters 6, 7 and 8 and explores both innovative developments and revisionary practices. In this context, the contribution made by the user/survivor movements is appraised and the impact of users/survivors repositioned as experts, is reviewed. In turn, the changing roles of workers and professionals within reconfigured organizational forms are interrogated and the opportunities and constraints incorporated within multi-disciplinary and multi-agency working are subject to critical scrutiny.

With regard to the content of specific chapters, in Chapter 2, the various understandings of mental health and the ways in which these understandings have influenced policy and practice, are critically appraised. This chapter explores a wide range of theoretical orientations which have been applied to mental distress. Rather than attention being paid to particular perspectives and adherents of these perspectives, there is a concentration on the work of a selection of commentators who accept that mental distress can be variously understood and responded to and who have put forward multi-faceted ways of exploring this contested area. The frameworks and analyses produced by Clare (1988), Pilgrim and Rogers (1999), Sayce (2000) and Horwitz (2002) are put forward as warranting further examination because all, in different ways, have engaged with a range of diverse models and conceptualizations. The critical appraisal of these multi-dimensional analyses is used to draw attention to three main themes which continue to inform the book as a whole. The first of these examines whether there are identifiable conditions or forms of behaviour which can be categorized in a particular way. This is in turn link to debates about social constructionism and social realism. The second is concerned, not so much with whether a condition is 'real' or 'constructed', but with how an individual associated with a condition or problem is responded to and the responses available. This is related to how a user/survivor is positioned and how users/survivors in turn can position themselves and others. The third theme explores how diagnosis and the medical confirmation of distress as an illness can be double-edged in that it can reassure and benignly explain the behaviour of 'patients' to themselves and others whilst also confirming vulnerability and the need for both 'care' and 'control'.

Chapter 3 provides an historical overview of mental health policy with emphasis placed on highlighting those prevailing themes which impact on the contemporary picture. In this chapter, the shifts and changes in thinking about mental well-being, mental health and illness are acknowledged, together with the continuing influence of concerns about risk and dangerousness. In particular the changes which have taken place since the decline of the asylums and the shift away from an ethos of institutionalization towards care in the community, are explored. Current mental health policy is located within the wider picture of health and social care and the development of a mixed economy of care, marked by the NHS and Community Care Act (1990). It is noted that many of the developments initiated by the Conservative government have remained in place since 1997 when the Labour government commenced its 'modernization' agenda. The obstacles to reform and the tensions inherent in this process are set out as a platform for further debate in Chapter 5.

Chapter 4 acknowledges the recognition that prejudice, stigma and fear have been and remain a significant part of the experience of people who have mental health difficulties. In this chapter the various challenges to prevailing views are identified. These include the impact of policies associated with community care and de-institutionalization, with the accompanying rise of consumer rights, user involvement and participation; the development of critical psychiatry and the survivor movement; and wider challenges to the oppression of minority and marginalized groups by means of anti-racist, anti-sexist movements and disability rights organizations. An important aspect of this discussion is to unravel the various dimensions relating to oppression and discrimination, especially with regard to ethnicity and gender, which underpin the broader picture. Methodological issues are considered as part of a review of the over-representation of black and minority ethnic groups in certain more controlling aspects of service provision and the concomitant under-representation of such groups in primary care services and therapeutic/support services (Fernando 1995; Sainsbury Centre for Mental Health [SCMH], 2002). Additionally, the gendered nature of mental health, which permeates throughout theoretical discussions, policy developments and practice, is examined (Prior 1999; Payne 1998; Wilton 1998). Recent initiatives in England concerning the needs of women and men from black and minority ethnic groups are also explored (Department of Health [DOH] 2002a; DOH 2003c).

Chapter 5 examines the contemporary policy and practice framework. In this context, the impact of *Modernising Mental Health Services: Safe, Sound and Supportive* (DOH 1998) is appraised and the influence of the *National*

Service Framework for Mental Health (DOH 1999a) and *The NHS Plan* (DOH 2000b), together with other legislative developments, are examined. The picture presented is that New Labour has energetically tackled entrenched problems in the field of mental health. They have set in motion a comprehensive system of clinical governance which incorporates a systematic setting of standards with milestones and performance indicators and monitoring processes. The importance of training and professional self-regulation has been emphasized and they are trying to address recognized shortfalls in provision and resources whilst asserting the value of 'joined-up' thinking and partnership working. They have taken steps to involve service users, paying particular attention to women and those from black and minority ethnic backgrounds, and measures have been introduced to safeguard the public and to foster the social inclusion of those with mental health problems by means of welfare-to-work policies, the Disability Discrimination Act 1995 and the 2005 proposals for a commission for equality and equal rights. It is argued that it is inevitable that such an ambitious programme will contain inbuilt tension, paradox and inconsistency. It is also contended that new policies or those which are presented as such are not introduced in a vacuum, but have to 'bed down' with those which have gone before. Again tension, paradox and inconsistency become inevitable as old policies, practices and cultures either form an explosive mix with the new or, to use an analogy drawn from geomorphology, provide a further layer with associated elevations, depressions and points of erosion. An examination of these areas, which include the opposing themes of managing risk and promoting social inclusion, the pull between local and centralized models of service delivery, the emphasis on evidence-based practice versus the tailoring of services to meet individual needs, and the various challenges posed to the prevailing mental health framework from those who have experience of mental distress, is also used as a means of constructively critiquing current policy.

Issues relating to users/survivors are considered throughout the book, but Chapter 6 takes forward some of the main themes. It explores the history and development of the survivor movement and considers the impact of this movement in the field of mental health. In particular, the development and application of the social model of disability, initially developed with regard to physical disability and subsequently related to mental illness, is explored. The notion of 'recovery' (Allott and Loganathan 2002), as a concept conceived of by survivors rather than by professionals, is appraised together with the recognition that there is a tendency for such developments to be integrated and diluted within mainstream policy. The increasing recruitment of people with experience of service use to work in mental health services is also reviewed together with the varied perspectives on involvement which include campaigning, the development of user-led services and involvement in current service developments. Related to the idea of an approach to recovery which 'aims to support an individual in their own personal development, building self-esteem, identity and finding a meaning-ful role in society' (Allott and Loganathan 2002: 4) is the concept of citizen-ship. This somewhat overused and variously defined concept is interrogated and the varying operational implications are scrutinized.

In this chapter it is clearly acknowledged that although there are areas of overlap, the interests of service users and carers have to be considered separately. Since the early 1990s, carers have featured prominently in government policies and their financial importance in terms of saved expen-diture on public services has been acknowledged. However, often 'carers' are regarded as a distinct entity with emphasis being placed on homogenous rather than on heterogeneous factors. This chapter looks at dimensions relating to gender, age, class and ethnicity and unpacks stereotypical assumptions. The various understandings of mental health held by these diverse groupings are also reviewed and the implications for policy and practice are appraised.

Chapter 7 takes an historical perspective across the various professional groups involved in mental health care, including psychiatry, nursing and social work. It focuses on the development of the respective roles and the boundaries between the various components of the workforce. The implica-tions of these roles for relationships between workers and those they are working with are explored as part of a discussion looking at the purpose and implications of what has historically been presented as a clear-cut, albeit dynamic, distinction. Similarly, the impact of recent policy and practice directives is examined. Key areas focused on include the changing organizational context of health and social care services as well as the shift-ing patterns of workforce configurations influenced by the drive towards occupational standards and competence frameworks (with an emphasis on a flexible and multi-skilled workforce, DOH 2000a; SCMH 2000). The increasing introduction of non-professionally aligned support workers in a variety of posts and settings is also considered within what may be seen as a move towards 'deprofessionalization', although the value placed on such workers by service users and carers is acknowledged (SCMH 1997; Burns et al 2001). This chapter raises a number of questions concerning the future of the mental health workforce including who is best equipped to deliver the range of services and interventions which are seen to be required. Related questions focus on: what future is there for traditional professional roles, are current developments paving the way for the introduction of a generic mental health worker, and what part can survivors/workers play in new organizational configurations?

Chapter 8 examines the changing structure of mental health services within the wider context of health and social care policy. The concepts of 'joined-up' thinking and partnership working which underpin current developments are reviewed in terms of their impact on the commissioning and delivery of services. These are examined in the context of the move towards greater collaboration between different agencies and the trend towards the structural integration of services in joint health and social care trusts (Hudson 2000). Additionally, consideration is given to the increasing level of compulsion in moving towards partnership, as specified by The *NHS Plan* (DOH 2000b). A further factor to be explored is the impact of primary care trusts which, in some areas, are increasingly involved in the provision of mental health services. Alongside developments within the statutory health and social care sector, this chapter also considers the impact of other initiatives within mental health care and the developmental opportunities which arise from health action zones, healthy living centres, neighbourhood renewal projects and local strategic partnerships. In particular, the opportunity to address the shortfall of services within historically under-resourced communities is appraised, noting the potential development of services for Asian women, African-Caribbean communities, Irish communities and ethnic elders.

Chapter 9, the concluding chapter, reviews and draws together the key points made in previous chapters. It summarizes the arguments and places the developments in an overall historical context and policy framework. In this, the tensions and contradictions inherent within both mental health policy and the wider context of health and social care are fully appraised. This chapter acknowledges the competing discourses which can influence and shape future developments. The importance of maintaining and extending principles associated with flexible, multiple and wide-ranging rather than uni-causal explanations of mental distress is highlighted together with an emphasis on meaningful social involvement, flexibility and choice.

CONCLUDING REMARKS

Policy and practice in the arena of mental health is changing rapidly. The growth of service user organizations, associated dissatisfaction with conventional treatments, the impetus derived from the growth of the radical psychiatry movement, charges of institutionalized racism and sexism, concerns about risk and public protection and issues relating to social care and professional practice, have all resulted in major upheavals. This book explores and examines the changing face of mental health in England and Wales and, where relevant, identifies international concerns. The impact of the pressures of globalization in this area is also considered. Throughout the book, the development of user/survivor involvement in research, understandings, policy and practice informs the discussion.

Theory, policy and tensions

2 Theoretical underpinnings

> No one person, no one body of 'experts' can claim a monopoly on madness.
> (Ussher 1991: 296).

As discussed in the Introduction, the way in which behaviour is interpreted, particularly forms of behaviour which appear to be unpredictable, or difficult to understand, or which indicate a loss of self-control and can be seen to threaten an individual's or other people's well-being and safety, all contribute to the identification of mental distress as a problem requiring action. Problem identification is mediated by class, gender, 'race', ethnicity, sexuality and disability. Porter (1991) opens his exploration of madness with a reputed quote from the Restoration playwright Nathaniel Lee. This remark 'They called me mad and I called them mad, and damn them, they outvoted me' (Porter 1991: 1) sardonically highlights the importance of weight of opinion and historically specific consensus views about acceptable and unacceptable ways of thinking and forms of behaviour. Ideologies, political doctrines, traditions, cultural practices and prevailing discourses all influence what is tolerated, what is not and how divergence or difference is responded to.[1]

Over time, understandings of mental health have been caught up in debates about reason, unreason, acceptable and unacceptable religious

---

1 With regard to the term 'discourse', Foucault (1981) used it to highlight the various ways in which power, language and institutional practices combine at historically specific points in time to determine modes of thought or conceptions of normality. An illustration can prove to be pertinent here. Accordingly, at one historical juncture in one particular culture, the pervasive understanding of a woman having a vision of the Virgin Mary could emphasize prophetic and authenticating aspects. In line with this 'dominant discourse', the woman herself could be viewed as one chosen by God to deliver his message and eventual sainthood may be assured. At different points in time, in different cultural and political circumstances, dominant interpretations could veer from heresy to religious fanaticism, to political incorrectness, to madness, with all having different implications for the individual concerned.

visions, manifestations and practices, 'scientific' findings and philosophical/social/psychological doctrines. Psychiatry, whose roots can be traced back to the sixteenth century, has been continually presented as 'objective' and as a way of scientifically understanding and treating disorders of the mind or emotions. This is despite psychiatry, like medicine, continuing to overturn and question preceding orthodoxies. There are many examples which could be used to illustrate this point. Fernando (1995) draws attention to the diagnostic category of 'Dysaesthesia Aethiopis' used by Cartwright in 1851, a reputable doctor of the time, to refer to a disease characterized by 'insensibility' of the skin and 'hebetude' of the mind. This was a condition claimed to afflict 'free Negroes'. Cartwright also famously described the diagnostic category of 'Drapetomania', a disease which caused slaves to run away. Maudsley (1887) saw a clear connection between masturbation and the onset of delusions and Charcot (1887–8) pointed to hysteria, particularly in women, as having a distinct physical cause. It is also notable that homosexuality was only excluded from the major classification system, the American Psychiatric Association's *Diagnostic and Statistical Manual of Mental Disorders*, third edition (DSM III), in 1980.

When reviewing approaches to mental health, a conventional approach is to look at specific disciplines and to explore psychiatric, psychological and sociological understandings. This has merit in that the differences between the understandings can clearly be highlighted and examined. However, there are also problems in that it is all too easy to give the impression that there is a broad consensus or homogeneity within discipline areas. In the same vein, similarities between understandings across the disciplines can be overlooked and the review can appear pedestrian and predictable. In order to avoid these pitfalls, this chapter will focus on a wide range of theoretical perspectives which have been applied to the field of mental distress. Rather than attention being paid to particular orientations and adherents of these orientations, there is a concentration on the work of a selection of commentators who accept that mental health/mental distress can be variously understood and responded to and who have posited various ways of going about this not inconsiderable task. Accordingly, it is contended that the frameworks produced by Clare (1988), Pilgrim and Rogers (1999), Sayce (2000) and Horwitz (2002) merit further exploration, not least because all grapple with a range of diverse conceptualizations.

The classic text by Clare (1988), entitled *Psychiatry in Dissent*, looks at models of 'mental illness' within psychiatry. Clare identifies four orientations. The first is the 'organic orientation' which views all mental illnesses as having an underlying physical pathology, even if the physical cause has not yet been identified. The second 'psychotherapeutic orientation' is primarily related to an emphasis on intrapsychic conflicts, mental mechanisms and the transference between analyst and analysand. Clare also incorporates the work of Thomas Szasz within this understanding. Szasz (1971) saw mental health difficulties resulting from 'problems with living' rather than diseases.

He emphasized that unless an individual had broken the law, in which case he or she should be liable to the usual penalties, it was up to the individual to decide whether she or he wanted therapeutic help or not. If she or he did, it was for that individual to enter into a voluntary and private contract with a therapist and to pay for services received. The third approach referred to by Clare is the 'sociotherapeutic approach'. Here, the contribution of environmental and social forces is prioritized. Accordingly, the mind/body dichotomy is reduced in importance and it is no longer the individual but the individual plus the social situation that becomes the object of the psychiatrist's concern. The fourth orientation Clare calls the 'medical model' and this is his preferred approach. He posits a broad version of a 'medical model', which incorporates aspects of all the models he has discussed. He says: 'The medical model, in short, takes into account not merely the symptom, syndrome, or disease, but the person who suffers, his personal and social situation, his biological, psychological and social status. The medical model, as applied to psychiatry, embodies the basis principle that every illness is the product of two factors – of environment working on the organism' (Clare 1988: 69).

Pilgrim and Rogers (1999) adopt a sociological perspective and take account of variables such as social class, gender, 'race', ethnicity and age. With regard to varying orientations, they focus on those perspectives 'outwith' sociology and include here the lay view; psychiatry; psychology and psychoanalysis; and the legal framework. In relation to those perspectives 'within' sociology they include social causation, societal reaction (labelling theory), critical theory, social constructivism and social realism.

This organization of understandings and responses is helpful and with regard to the first grouping, those outwith sociology, Pilgrim and Rogers draw attention to the 'certain persuasiveness' of each together with inbuilt 'credibility' problems. They highlight the ways in which illness models and legal frameworks focus on discontinuity, that is, an individual either has a recognizable condition or she or he does not, whilst other perspectives included in this grouping emphasize continuity, which can be visualized as a roller-coaster transition between mental health and mental ill-health. This is particularly the case with regard to psychoanalytical orientations.

At this point before moving on to look at those orientations 'within' sociology, given their influence, it is useful to provide a brief overview of psychological orientations, particularly those based on psychoanalytic/psychotherapeutic understandings and learning theory, or as Pilgrim and Rogers (1999) describe the latter, 'the presence of specific behaviours' and 'distorted cognitions' (Pilgrim and Rogers 1999: 8–9).

Psychoanalysis originated with Freud and his orientation was primarily biological. This is seen particularly in his portrayal of instincts. In terms of therapy, there is a clear focus on the joint aims of life being love and work. In order to maximize well-being, Freud maintained that the ego needs the energy of the libido to draw upon as energy is wasted if libidinous impulses are repressed. Patterson (1986) regards the objectives of psychoanalysis as being the freeing of healthy impulses, the strengthening of reality-based ego functioning[2] and altering the contents of the superego (conscience, social and parental sanction) to ensure it is not overly punitive.

There are many variations of psychoanalysis and forms of psychotherapy (for example, Adler, Fromm, Jung, Erikson, Alexander, Klein). Despite some similarities and many differences, all offer a distinctive all-embracing conceptual/diagnostic/treatment continuum in relation to mental health and ill-health and all analyse and interpret behaviour in accordance with this framework.

Learning theory includes behavioural therapy, social learning such as 'Learned Helplessness' (Seligman 1975) and cognitive behaviour therapy. Although there are many very different approaches, all rest on the premise that all behaviour is learned and can consequently be 'unlearned'. Emphasis is placed on eradicating problematic behaviours and/or thought processes, rather than on how specific behaviours or 'faulty thinking' arose in the first place. Treatment processes draw from experimentally established principles and procedures and are controlled, systematic and measured. Like psycho-analytical orientations, conceptual frameworks and treatment programmes are self-referential and inclusive.

Pilgrim and Rogers (1999) maintain that all these outwith understandings, despite claims of objectivity and universality, can be seen to be value-laden, incorporating prevailing views and assumptions. They contend that none can be privileged over another and assert: 'What we have is a fragmented set of perspectives, divided internally and from one another, which occasionally enter the same world of discourse' (1999: 11).

In their discussion of those orientations 'within' sociology, Pilgrim and Rogers (1999) emphasize the ways in which the broad discipline of sociology has on the one hand focused on identifying the causes of mental illness and on the other has established competing ways of conceptualizing abnormality. Social causation is described as a way of looking at mental health that accepts diagnostic categories, but which investigates those social situations and stress factors most commonly associated with particular conditions. The famous study by Brown and Harris (1978) which looks at the social origins of depression (referred to in more detail in Chapter 4), is cited as adopting a social causation perspective. This can also be seen to be an approach favoured by governments where currently addressing social exclusion is regarded as a precursor, not only of tackling mental health problems, but also of crime, unemployment, substance abuse and ill-health generally.

---

2 The strengthening of reality-based ego functioning includes widening the perception of the ego (that part of the id which has been influenced by the external world) so that it approves more of the id. The inner inherited psychic world orientated towards the satisfaction of instinctual needs by means of the pleasure principle. It is also the location of the unconscious.

With regard to different ways of conceptualizing abnormality, Pilgrim and Rogers (1999) focus on four main frameworks. These are societal reaction or labelling theory, critical theory, social constructivism or social constructionism and critical realism. Given the significance of these it is useful briefly to review broad definitions of these orientations.

Labelling theory was particularly popular in the late 1960s and early 1970s and is associated with the movement in sociology known as symbolic interactionism. It is popularly viewed as a way of looking at how an individual initially acquires a label and then at how individuality can be subsumed into that label. However, Scheff (1966), one of the prime proponents of this approach, focused on how deviance from expected roles is initially denied by those close to an individual (primary deviance) and then at how, once a person acquires a label, subsequent behaviour is interpreted in accordance with that deviant role or label (secondary deviance).

Critical theory, in turn, is associated with the work of the Frankfurt Institute of Social Research founded in 1923 which became famously known as the Frankfurt School. Although the work of those associated with this school has been wide-ranging, there is a general focus on the relationship between socio-economic structures and the inner psyches of individuals. Pilgrim and Rogers (1999) see critical theory as relevant to sociological conceptualizations of mental health because of the various ways in which proponents have connected the psyche and society.

Social constructivism or social constructionism has many interpretations and this is an area which will be referred to later in this chapter. However, Pilgrim and Rogers (1999) provide a working definition which gives a broad overview of commonalities. They state:

> A central assumption within this broad approach is that reality is not self evident, stable and waiting to be discovered, but instead is a product of human activity. In this broad sense all versions of social constructivism can be identified as a reaction against positivism and naïve realism.
>
> (Pilgrim and Rogers 1999: 18)

The orientation which Pilgrim and Rogers (1999) personally adhere to is that of social realism. This they describe as an approach which draws from, but also critically appraises, other approaches. There is an emphasis on critiquing particular discourses in the field of mental health, but this is linked to an acknowledgement of the existence of an external reality and to an acceptance that some aspects of mental ill-health, for example, forms of dementia, have a material cause.

Sayce (2000) adopts a social orientation and is primarily concerned with citizenship for users/survivors becoming a reality and upon overcoming discrimination and social exclusion. She wants movement to take place 'beyond' community care services so that users/survivors can both contribute to and be included in society (2000: 36). However, she is also mindful that alternative movement towards ever greater control and social exclusion remains an ongoing possibility.

Sayce (2000) examines a number of what she terms 'anti-stigma' approaches to mental health problems. The first is the 'Brain Disease Model'. Here possible social and familial influences give way to a focus on the organic brain. Accordingly, mental health becomes a brain disease, an illness like any other caused by biological and/or biochemical malfunctioning and influenced by genetic inheritance. In turn, responsibility for illness and actions is removed from the individual, their family and their socio-economic circumstances. The physical condition is also, by association, treatable by physical means.

However, Sayce (2000) pertinently states that: 'History gives little comfort to those who believe that if only the public knew that mentally ill people "could not help it", they would readily come to respect and value them' (2000: 93). She highlights how genetic arguments can be used to justify a variety of contradictory positions from 'no fault' assertions, to arguments that mental ill-health is a sign of genetic inferiority that should be eradicated. She further maintains that: 'Removing responsibility from people is to deny their humanity. It leads to the most paternalistic and abusive tendencies of welfare provision' (2000: 95). She asserts a little later: 'Additionally, the power of the vested interests pursuing this model means other messages, especially those promoted by users/survivors themselves, are easily eclipsed' (2000: 99).

The second 'anti-stigma' approach which Sayce appraises is that which she terms the 'Individual Growth Model'. This model views mental health and mental ill-health as part of a continuum, with mental health and well-being at one end of a fluid line and mental ill-health at the other. The application of this model ensures that individuals retain responsibility for their actions, but in so doing they retain responsibility for their health and for their recovery or non-recovery. As she points out, it blurs distinctions between mental health and mental ill-health, but at the cost of ignoring structural factors both in relation to causation and with regard to gaining inclusion as full citizens.

The 'Libertarian Model' is the third model reviewed. This revolves around campaigns for equal rights and responsibilities for those with mental health problems. This approach rejects compulsory treatment and coercion in any form. It also dismisses the taking of action on the basis of perceived or assessed risk. It has a clear message, which appears to draw from the work of Thomas Szasz (1971) in categorically rejecting specific mental health provision for those perceived as mentally ill. If an individual has committed a criminal act, then, the argument goes, he or she should be subject to the penalties of the criminal law. Sayce commends the role that proponents of this model have played in drawing attention to abuses and in campaigning to limit and end compulsory treatment, but maintains that 'getting the state off users' backs does not seem, to many users/survivors in Britain or the USA, to be a sufficient strategy' (2000: 128). She also questions whether the power base of supporters is strong enough for this model to ever achieve a position of dominance.

The 'Disability Inclusion' model is the fourth approach which Sayce appraises. This is the model which Sayce personally favours and the one which she believes has the greatest potential to tackle 'stigma' and discrimination. This model is clearly linked to the civil rights agenda of the disability movement. Sayce acknowledges that not all users/survivors want to establish a connection with the disability movement and that there are concerns relating to the specific ways in which those with mental health problems are responded to. However, she argues that the tackling of discriminatory social barriers is a platform which should be broadly embraced and which also leaves room for specific challenges to be separately addressed.

Horwitz (2002) adheres to a broadly sociological perspective and views mental health in a very different way. He takes an historical journey through the twentieth century, comparing and contrasting what he calls 'dynamic psychiatry', which he sees as being about uncovering the intrapsychic conflicts that lie beneath manifest symptoms, and 'diagnostic psychiatry', which is about the diagnosis and treatment of symptom-based diseases. He argues that in America, particularly during the first two thirds of the twentieth century, dynamic psychiatry expanded definitions of the pathological from the psychoses to a range of what he describes as 'indeterminate manifestations of underlying unconscious mechanisms' (2002: 208). He maintains that the 'loose classifications' of dynamic psychiatry were appropriate during a period when mental health professionals did not need a rationalized quantitative system of thought about mental disorder, but that once professional, economic and organizational circumstances changed, the approach to psychiatry had to change also. He remarks: 'If psychiatrists were to be treated as "real" physicians, then they needed to treat "real" diseases' (2002: 210). He argues that disease-based classification systems such as DSM III (American Psychiatric Association 1980) or its fourth edition DSM IV (American Psychiatric Association 1994) came to dominate from the late 1970s onwards as a result of intraprofessional concerns, but also because of the interest of the pharmaceutical industry. Like Sayce (2000), he emphasizes how a disease-based model reduces stigma for families and individuals. He asserts that a generalized acceptance, at the beginning of the twenty-first century, of mental illnesses as disease entities has resulted 'less from advances in the scientific understanding of mental disorder that disease classifications have brought about than from the many advantages these classifications have for a variety of professional and lay groups' (2002: 213).

However, Horwitz sees a social constructionist perspective as being limited. He maintains that 'While mental illnesses are social constructions, *something* is being constructed' (2002: 229). Although he believes that social constructionist perspectives can explain how a medicalized categorical system of mental illness emerged and persisted through a particular historical era, he does not accept that such perspectives can evaluate the adequacy of a classification system such as DSM III (American Psychiatric Association 1980) or DSM IV (American Psychiatric Association 1994). He claims that it is necessary to use criteria which stem from outside a social constructionist perspective to judge the validity of classification systems. In this respect the questions he poses are first whether valid mental disorder exists and second whether a condition can be usefully viewed as a disease. Accordingly, Horwitz regards the psychoses as being amenable to the disease model of diagnostic psychiatry, but questions whether non-psychotic disorders, such as those linked to stress or forms of social deviance that violate social norms of right and wrong conduct, should attract mental health labels. He concludes:

> Constructing some kinds of disturbed human behaviour as diseases fits some conditions better than others. Those who are concerned with mental health and illness should not assume either that mental illness labels are appropriate whenever they are applied or that they are never appropriate. Instead, they should strive to specify when people have internal dysfunctions or, alternatively, when they are making normal responses to the social situations in which they find themselves. Ultimately, they need to consider when restoring normality is best accomplished by changing individuals and when it is best done by transforming social conditions.
>
> (Horwitz 2002: 229)

All of the authors whose conceptualizations are outlined above clearly question taken-for-granted assumptions about mental health. None can be taken as representative of their field or discipline, but all by means of their analysis contribute to understandings of mental distress which draw attention to the variety and diversity of the ontological and epistemological perspectives which operate. However, all orientations, even those as wide-ranging as those outlined, in order to prevent inflexibility in interpretation need to be subject to constructive critique. With regard to Clare (1988), his project is clearly to formulate an all-embracing, inclusive medical model. However, just as prioritization of risk can result in an understanding of mental distress where all other factors become moulded around this central tenet, so too can a 'medical model', as defined by Anthony Clare, become so inclusive that social and environmental orientations, for example, lose their critical edge and become yet another smooth cog supporting the operation of a well-oiled, yet specifically orientated machine. Inclusivity, with regard to theoretical perspectives, can neutralize critique and become counterproductive. Sayce too, in understandably trying to strengthen the political platform for the survivor/user movement, tries to smooth jagged edges and, by implication, to subsume issues of difference and diversity. This is a critique that can be levelled at the disability movement. It can also be asserted that the incorporation of users/survivors into existing organizational planning forums can easily erode and neutralize the original hard-edged messages born of direct and mediated experience. In certain contexts user/survivor perspectives can be watered down, tensions ameliorated and areas of conflict smoothed over.

Pilgrim and Rogers (1999) and also Horwitz (2002) wrestle with analyses that draw from social constructionism and critical theory. Both acknowledge the part played by prevailing power/knowledge paradigms and values in constructing the various ways in which mental distress is understood, but both, in different ways, distance themselves from relativism. Pilgrim and Rogers do this by embracing social realism, and Horwitz by making it clear that, notwithstanding the influence of social constructionism, *something* is being constructed.

However, given these points of critique, the multi-dimensional analyses presented by Clare (1988), Pilgrim and Rogers (1999), Sayce (2000) and Horwitz (2002) have proved influential in the development of three broad overlapping themes presented in this book. The first of these explores whether there are identifiable conditions or forms of behaviour which can be categorized and responded to in a particular way. This theme can be associated with the debates about social constructionism and social realism with linkages to poststructuralist and structuralist paradigms. The second focuses not so much on whether a condition is 'real' or 'constructed', but on how an individual associated with a condition or problem is responded to and the responses available to her or him. Alternatively this could be looked at in terms of how a user/survivor is both positioned and how he or she in turn can position both themselves and others. The third relates to how diagnosis and confirmation of illness can be double-edged in that it can reassure and benignly explain the behaviour of 'patients' to themselves and family members whilst also confirming vulnerability and the need for both 'care' and 'control'.

With regard to the first theme, the work of Foucault has made a significant if complex contribution. In his early work he focused on the powers of surveillance and used the example of Bentham's panopticon, a design aimed at unidirectional, maximum surveillance to draw attention to the invasive impact of 'the gaze'. He explored the operation of power and coined the label 'eventalization' to draw attention to events being contingent rather than inevitable. His method was inductive in that he started out with an event such as the identification and treatment of 'mad' people and worked backwards, looking at how definitions and categorizations were established (Foucault 1981: 6). Foucault associated all of these with the operation of power and regarded power and knowledge frameworks as being indivisible. He viewed power as operating within everyday social practices. He argued that although dominant discourses are created at specific points in time by particular ways of thinking, supported in turn by the power of governments and large institutions, the process is far from straightforward. He maintained that those discourses which come to dominate arise from what is already there, with overriding institutional sanction operating as a means of legitimizing certain social practices. According to this analysis, for example, the separation of the 'deserving' from the 'undeserving' poor in the 1830s by means of the workhouse system would have developed from everyday discursive practices and prejudices, before being legitimized by legislation and policy.

Foucault wanted to know how power manifested in social practices is exercised through the interplay of discourses. Accordingly, he focused on how, for example, dividing practices could not only achieve a position of dominance in a particular historical period, separating 'the mad' from 'the sane', but could also be seen to be scientific and objective. Foucault also critiqued the power of experts and drew attention to how various therapeutic techniques or 'psy complexes' could be used to control subjects. He further identified a process which resulted in the formation of what he called 'docile bodies'. Here, over time individuals subjected to particular forms of regulation, come to monitor and control their own behaviour in order to fit the requirements of a particular social setting. This creates 'docile bodies' and results in the behaviour of others being standardized through direct and, equally influential, indirect means.

Overall, there can be seen to be a range of social constructionist approaches and all vary considerably (Burr 1995). However, all to differing degrees highlight the importance of language, meaning and context. Social reality is seen to be constructed in accordance with how language is used and how meanings are attached in situational and historically specific contexts. Derrida (1978) contended that meaning could never be fixed and he maintained that it must always be viewed as provisional. Inherent within this interpretation is the view that the person or people uttering a sound or producing a written image are immaterial to the creation of meaning. Derrida's analysis has been charged with introducing a form of relativism which makes it impossible to cite any external legitimating authority for any perspective and with making it impossible to weight one claim over another (e.g., Di Stefano 1990; Brodrib 1992; Jackson 1992; Busfield 1996). However, other writers, particularly those who have engaged with postmodern feminism, have drawn from Derrida, Foucault and postmodernist influences to engage in 'a more complex inquiry into the relationship between identity, agency and welfare discourses, and how these combine in different ways to shape the materiality of people's lives' (Williams 1994: 14–15). Similarly, Fraser and Nicholson (1993) look to locate social criticism within comparative, historically, temporally and culturally specific accounts and to reject ahistorical, legitimating and transcendental discourse.[3]

---

3 See Fawcett (2000) for a wider discussion of these orientations.

In relation to the second theme, it is clear that clinical paradigms are often unhelpfully set against more socially orientated frameworks which focus on removing stigma, stressing citizenship rights and promoting a broader-based response to mental distress. There are also approaches which celebrate difference and uniqueness and look for new ways of giving voice to unusual and distinctive experiences. Disparate organizations such as Mad Pride and the Hearing Voices network adopt this stance. This latter network has been built up around the work of Marius Romme and Sandra Escher. In a ground-breaking book entitled *Accepting Voices* published in 1993, Romme and Escher positively revalued hearing voices and researched ways of coping with voices that were not drug-related. They discovered a number of people who said that they heard voices but had never used psychiatric services. Although Romme and Escher acknowledge that hearing voices can be a problem for some, Escher, Romme and Buiks (1998), following further work with children, maintained that the 'normalization' of voice hearing clearly helps individuals cope and achieve their desired goals without additional intervention. They accept that for some the hearing of voices might be a problem with this depending on the negative or positive nature of the voices. However, they maintain that not every problem which involves voice hearing is an illness and that there are alternatives to drug treatments. In this context, Wilson and Beresford (2002) draw attention to how, within conventional practice, individual experiences are easily moulded to fit classificatory frameworks and how a mental health diagnosis serves both to nullify personal aspirations and to influence how an individual is responded to for the rest of his or her life.

This theme highlights the importance of different perspectives and understandings and the utility of having a range of flexible frameworks so that each person's difficulties can be located within a structure and an associated explanatory frame that proves most helpful at that particular point in time. In relation to this theme, two examples can be given. One clearly relates to 'hearing voices'. The recognition that this may or may not be a problem for a particular individual is perhaps an important initial acknowledgement in its own right. If it is perceived to be a problem, an individual may feel more comfortable within a frame of reference that views hearing voices as a symptom of an illness which is amenable to pharmaceutical treatment. Here, an individual may also want to produce an advance directive stating the action he or she would want taking should they lose control. If a diagnosis/illness/treatment model is not one that appears helpful, then other support systems such as Hearing Voices or other networks may enable the individual to cope with problematic voices. In turn, however the difficulty is understood, user or survivor groups may prove useful in that they provide a forum for sharing experiences and campaigning for change in mutually identified areas. Another example relates to 'depression'. If an individual perceives this as a problem which she or he requires help with, it may be useful for this to be viewed as an illness with associated treatment and support facilities. Alternatively a spiritual interpretation may be appropriate, or forms of therapeutic intervention, such as psychoanalysis or cognitive behaviour therapy, or support provided by user/survivor groups.

In the field of mental health, the pendulum periodically swings between the protection of the public and the individual needs and rights of a person experiencing mental distress. Currently, given a number of high-profile homicides and media outrage,[4] policy and practice have focused firmly on the protection of the public and risk assessment is a major part of any assessment/diagnosis frame. This can lead to inflexibility and rigidity, with compliance being emphasized over individual preferences. The efficacy of this response is discussed in more detail in Chapters 4, 5 and 7, and the point to be made at this stage relates to the ways in which the imposition of a particular interpretation, a 'one size fits all approach', can result in conceptual and practical limitations and constraints and to other aspects being obscured.

Overall, this second theme uses the various perspectives as points of critique and as a means of positively and constructively informing debates. However, it is also one which appraises but also privileges the ways in which users/survivors can position themselves as well as interrogating the ways in which, in accordance with prevailing dominant and not so dominant discourses, they can be positioned.

With regard to the third theme, the orientation utilized in this book accepts that for both individuals and carers, there can be advantages associated with a medicalized diagnosis and treatment framework. As Sayce (2000) comments, pharmaceutical companies are major players in this area and fund major publicity campaigns stressing, for example, that 'depression' is an illness which can be straightforwardly treated by advances in pharmacology. Explanations of violent and dramatic events, such as an estranged husband killing his wife and children, are made more palatable if a label of mental illness can be attached. The event then becomes tragic, but responsible others enter the frame. Social workers, health professionals and the police are called to account for not recognizing the 'symptoms' and doing something about it. This prevents the dangerous acknowledgement that such behaviour, given a particular set of circumstances, is something that all of us are capable of when emotions are running high and accustomed personal power and control regimes are threatened. However, it is

---

4 For example, the killing of Isabel Schwartz by a former social work client Sharon Campbell in 1984; Michael Buchanan who in 1992 following discharge from hospital killed a stranger in a car park; the stabbing of Jonathan Zito by Christopher Clunis in 1992; the death of Jonathan Newby brought about by John Rous; the attack on Georgina Robinson by Andrew Robinson in 1993; the stabbing of Bryan Bennet by Stephen Laudat in 1994; and the killing by Kenneth Gray of his mother in 1995. The point that is made is that tragic though these incidents are, compared to other forms of homicide the incidence is extremely small.

also a means of explanation that promotes the construction of the 'other'. As Fawcett and Hearn (2004) point out, the notion of 'Otherness' is both complex and has a complex history. Otherness has been ascribed on the basis of class, 'race', gender, ethnicity, disability and 'non-Westernness', with particular forms of 'Otherness' being prioritized at different points in time. 'Otherness' (or forms of Otherness) can be identified in relation to social power relations and discursive formulations. The construction of the 'other' is used to legitimize forms of behaviour and power imbalances which would be deemed unacceptable without the use of this form of distancing. However, it is also worthy of note that being positioned as 'other' can be used as a means of drawing attention to and revaluing a devalued construction. This can be seen in the disability literature in the ways that terms such as 'cripple' have been used by those with impairments to challenge and to positively appropriate negative labels. In this way, this theme has very clear links with the second theme discussed above and, throughout this book, notions of 'otherness' in terms of creation and response will continue to be appraised.

CONCLUDING REMARKS

The three themes discussed in this chapter are clearly interrelated. They derive from a range of sources and influence the ontological and epistemological perspectives adopted in this book. These themes build on the different ways in which mental health or mental distress can be understood and take account of how a range (and a far from exhaustive range) of critical analysts have both deconstructed and constructed conceptual paradigms.

In this chapter, emphasis has been placed on highlighting that there are many ways of understanding and responding to individual and group manifestations of mental distress. It has also been maintained that despite claims to objectivity and factual correctness, nothing can be regarded as fixed and immutable. This is not to say that individuals do not lose control and behave in ways which are difficult for others to understand and that factors such as genetics, chemical imbalances, personal, social and environmental factors do not play a contributory role. However, rather than specific explanations being emphasized, this chapter has focused on exploring the various understandings and associated responses. Accordingly, prominence has been given to the critical interrogation of dominant frameworks. This is not to highlight one approach or direction and to attribute value to it, but to critically and constructively investigate what is going on, the theoretical underpinnings and the associated implications for all stakeholders. Undeniably, clinical understandings which highlight aspects relating to health and define problems as illnesses with symptoms which can be categorized and treated predominantly, but not exclusively, with drug and physical treatments, currently hold a position of dominance. This is the view supported by the government and reinforced by legislation and policy. From an international perspective, it is also the dominant way of understanding mental distress. As mentioned in the Introduction, increasing globalization has been associated with the further standardization of ideas, policies and practices. However, as Fook (2002) points out, debates about the economic and political consequences of globalization sit side by side with postmodern forms of theorizing which emphasize relativity, fragmentation, the difficulty of privileging any particular opinion, including that of the 'expert', and the overall dissolution of the certainties of modernism. Fawcett and Featherstone (1996) look at how the management of current welfare services is characterized by attempts to reproduce the large certainties or the taken-for-granted 'truths' of modernism, as 'small certainties' (i.e. performance targets, the concretization of professional tasks, the efficacy of risk assessment based on diagnostic categories and so on) that can be reimposed in a postmodern age. In this book, therefore, current certainties such as the key tenets of the prevailing mental health system are interrogated along with those perspectives which can be considered to be less well defined in the public consciousness and more marginally supported in terms of resources.

3 The historical policy framework

To define true madness
What is't but to be nothing else but mad?

(Hamlet, Act II, Sc.ii, l. 93)

In this chapter a historical overview of mental health policy is provided with particular emphasis being placed on those continuing themes which impact on the contemporary picture. This acknowledges the shifts and changes in thinking about mental health and illness as well as the continuing influence of concerns about risk and dangerousness. In particular the changes which have taken place since the decline of the asylums and the shift away from an ethos of institutionalization towards care in the community are explored.

THE HISTORICAL CONTEXT

A review of policy, and mental health policy in particular, is by no means straightforward. Whilst a historical perspective may shed light on the precursors of contemporary developments and issues, this in itself cannot be undertaken in isolation from wider questions and concerns. In particular a number of questions arise which require further attention if the complexities and nuances of mental health policy are to be acknowledged. These include the conceptualization, principles and boundaries of health and social policy and some recognition of the constantly shifting dynamics which underpin change as well as a questioning of the modernist endeavour towards relentless progress. Mental health policy needs to be identified as confusing, ambiguous and contradictory territory, the mapping of which is unlikely to be accurate and the navigation of which may need to be guided by clear perspectives and points for orientation.

The first section of this chapter aims to set some clear signposts which will assist the readers in finding their way through and making sense of the landscape. These will consider, in turn, the range of perspectives concerning what is meant by health and social policy, state welfare and the welfare state; the relationship between policy and the wider social and economic context; the interplay of factors concerning medicine and in particular psychiatry; and finally the meaning of 'mental health' within any point of time or space/geography. Additionally, it will be important to take a critical view of change and to examine the extent to which apparent shifts in thinking and policy reflect fundamental second order change or are merely indicative of first order change in the dynamics of power and inequality. Shifts of power within multi-disciplinary working or the notion of service user involvement can be used as examples here.

This mapping exercise will provide a framework for an historical overview of mental health policy which forms the second element of this chapter. Whilst a detailed history will be beyond the scope of this book, this will provide a backdrop for contemporary developments, recognizing that the legacy of the past provides one route into an understanding of the complexities of the present.

HEALTH AND SOCIAL POLICY, STATE WELFARE AND THE WELFARE STATE

Mental health policy can only be understood as one strand within the wider health and social care context and lies at the interface of what is increasingly seen as a continuous spectrum of policy and related services and practices. The origins and development of policy as a concept also have to be placed in the context of the historical development of the nation state, prior to which the arrangements for the care of those deemed to be vulnerable were local, unsystematic and provided within a nexus of relationships based on a rural agrarian economy.

Lewis (2000) refers to social policy as containing a range of distinct meanings; these include an understanding of government policies 'intended to improve the social well-being or welfare of citizens' (Lewis 2000: 4) and a broader definition which includes issues of policing, crime, criminal justice and the recognition that the care and well-being of citizens may also be balanced by issues of control and regulation. An additional perspective here also concerns the extent to which social policy is seen to concern itself primarily with the 'public' rather than the 'private', emphasizing the systematic, institutionalized and cash-dependent provision of support and services as opposed to the domestic and familial delivery of care which by its nature highlights the differential role played by women and men. Lewis also questions whether only government policies are within the remit of social policy given the role played by other social institutions including international bodies. For example, certain recent changes in policy and practice in Britain owe their introduction to initiatives driven within the European Union rather than by national government. At a more subtle level it is also possible to identify shifts and changes of policy influenced by events and developments outside of national boundaries and the existence of what might be termed 'policy-borrowing' within a global rather than a national perspective. There is also evidence of increasing convergence between historically separate systems (Rochefort and Goering 1998). Dominelli also refers to globalization as a 'macro-level phenomenon with micro-level implications' in terms of the need to locate social policy within this wider context (2002: 45).

The first meaning is embedded in a history of social administration exemplified by Titmuss (1963) who also recognized the need to examine social policy within the wider picture of social and economic conditions, social change and social relations, thus raising issues of inequality and power. Williams (1994, quoted in D Taylor 1996) similarly highlights that welfare policies are underpinned by social relationships including class, race, gender, sexuality, disability and age and that these may be contested. Taylor (1996) points out that social policy plays a part in 'enabling or disabling' social participation and draws attention to the way in which discrimination and oppression underpin welfare outcomes. However, access to services and support may be at the cost of control or regulation for certain groups distinguished by gendered or racialized boundaries.

The concept of the welfare state is closely allied to notions of social policy although Goodwin and Mitchell (2000) comment that it 'is not one thing but many and both its foundation and manifestation are many and varied' (2000: ix). However, it is generally understood to be characterized by systematic state concern for the welfare of people who might otherwise lack basic necessities, a definition which implicitly relates to issues concerning levels of need and the identification of those who are deemed to lack the 'basic necessities'. A further refinement of this definition also links the notion of the welfare state to particular economic and political regimes, specifically recognizing the relationship of the welfare state to capitalism and social democracy. This highlights differing concepts of need and *purpose* in terms of the beneficiaries of social interventions who may not necessarily be confined to those in receipt of any particular service. For example, a Marxist analysis suggests that, whilst social interventions may be necessary to maintain the well-being of the working classes at a sufficient level to ensure their productivity within a capitalist economy, meeting the real needs of the working classes is not viewed as being compatible with the interests of the capitalist market economy. Pierson (1998) also draws attention to the influence of societal changes in the development of the welfare state including the impact of industrialization, increasing population and demographic changes, the growth of nation states and accompanying notions of political democracy and citizenship (1998).

To relate some of these issues more specifically to mental health policy it may be helpful to explore the following questions: what are the key features associated with the development of mental health services; to what extent are these related to changing concepts of mental illness over broad historical periods and how do these relate to changing social and economic conditions?

Additionally, the question of how to understand mental health policy in relation to the issue of need and the extent to which this is for the general benefit of society or those individuals most directly affected in terms of their own health, also requires consideration. Allied to this is the importance of considering the ways in which mental health policy is underpinned by issues of social inequality and differential experiences mediated by race, gender, age, etc., and the extent to which these will affect an understanding of policy in terms of care or control and regulation.

THE RELATIONSHIP BETWEEN POLICY AND THE WIDER SOCIAL AND ECONOMIC CONTEXT

Historically, social policy is associated with the development of the nation state with the accompanying rise of a centralized infrastructure and government and an economy increasingly associated with trade and commerce. Prior to this period, life in Britain was characterized by an agrarian and rural economy where authority rested with the Church and local feudal lords, the latter offering limited protection in return for use of the land. The main providers of care for the sick and needy at this time were primarily the Church, including the monasteries. Financial support in the form of almsgiving, regarded as a form of spiritual insurance, provided for the setting up of almshouses and hospices as early forms of institutional care. Hospitals such as St Bartholomew's and St Thomas's in London were founded in 1123 and 1200 respectively. Bethlem Priory was established in 1247 although it did not initially undertake the care of the mentally distressed. These were accompanied by an underpinning belief in the value of charitable service and donations, as well as an understanding of sickness which rested on explanations which either recognized divine retribution or the work of the devil in causing illness.

In England the fifteenth century broadly represented the beginning of a centralized monarchy and a decrease in internal conflict and warfare which enabled the development of trade and commerce. The period of the Renaissance and the Reformation also paved the way for the scientific 'revolution' and the beginnings of the rise of medicine as a profession. Progress and advancement, however, were not to the benefit of all sections of society and the social 'costs' of the beginnings of urbanization and a money economy included increased destitution and vagrancy. This eventually resulted in the Elizabethan Poor Law.

THE INTERPLAY OF FACTORS CONCERNING MEDICINE AND IN PARTICULAR PSYCHIATRY

In relation to health care, mental health policy also needs to be located within the development of medicine and psychiatry at a particular historical juncture. The prevailing discourse in pre-industrial Britain concerned the understanding of illness and disease in terms of religion, the work of the devil or divine retribution. Alternative approaches, including the role of folk healers and herbalists, who were predominantly women, were at times strongly challenged in the form of witch hunts and executions (Ehrenreich and English 1979). At the same time folk healers and herbalists continued to provide a complementary system of care in which the administration of treatments and herbal remedies was accompanied by the markers of ritual healing, including recourse to both pagan and Christian practices such as the healing power of saints and the use of relics (Stacey 1988). The rise of the nation state, the shift from a feudal to a monetary economy and the development of the Renaissance and the Reformation were closely associated with a scientific revolution which linked exploration and discovery with the progressive modernist project. In relation to health care this has ultimately accorded privilege to biomedicine, despite the continuation and, to some extent, growing popularity of complementary approaches such as homeopathy, and an increasing recognition of other perspectives such as reflexology.

Parker et al (1995) draw on Foucault's suggestion that it is only after the fifteenth century that the notion of 'madness' was seen as a spectre to be feared alongside death, and became a preoccupation to replace leprosy and that "the mad" then filled the space that was opened up by the closure of the leprosaria at the end of the Middle Ages' (1995: 6). This then marked the beginning of a period of confinement which reached its peak with the development of the asylums and which only latterly was understood within a paradigm of care for the sick rather than confinement of the disorderly and deviant. This development itself needs to be considered within the context of the period of industrialization.

INDUSTRIALIZATION AND THE GROWTH OF THE ASYLUMS

Whilst the period of the Industrial Revolution is generally dated between 1760 and 1830 (Midwinter 1994), it is possible to locate this in a wider time-frame during which period a number of developments influenced social policy in general and issues of mental health and illness in particular. The social and economic environment of this time was characterized by the introduction of a manufacturing industry centred on the factory rather than the domestic setting, an increase in urbanization as the demands of the factory system and trade required a move away from small dispersed settlements focused around the demands of agriculture and local, self-sufficient communities, a rapidly growing population. From a population of 1.5 million in 1066, the population of England and Wales increased to 5.5 million in 1700 and then to 13 million by 1831. Furthermore it is estimated that in 1831, there were a total of 1.5 million paupers, approximately 1/40 of the population (Midwinter 1994).

Economic and social pressures in the aftermath of the Napoleonic Wars including unemployment and a concern that outdoor relief, involving payments to the poor living in their own homes, was increasingly costly, culminated in the Poor Law Amendment Act of 1834. This effectively paved the way for the establishment in all areas of workhouses, each overseen by a board of guardians underpinned by a belief that the receipt of financial support should be made as uncomfortable as possible to deter the 'undeserving'. As a consequence, the beginning of the nineteenth century saw an increase in workhouses representing an increasing shift from a domestic to an institutional ethos of care and by 1847 there were 707 workhouses with 200,000 places.

The demands of urban life included the need to deal with poor and inadequate housing and insanitary conditions and led to an increasing interest in issues of public health and a recognition of the negative impact of poor and overcrowded living conditions. Disease and malnutrition were widespread and reflected in high mortality rates with 25% of all children not living beyond the age of seventeen. The 1848 Public Health Act focused attention on the creation of drainage and sewage systems and the provision of clean water. Alongside the concern with public health this period also saw the 1858 Medical Act which legitimized the profession of medicine and the growth of nursing, made increasingly respectable by the endeavours of Florence Nightingale in the Crimean War (1854–6) and Mary Seacole both in the war and elsewhere. The work of Pasteur and Koch after 1860 also emphasized an increase in medical knowledge which in turn had important implications for health care.

THE GROWTH AND DECLINE OF THE ASYLUMS

Alongside these wider changes in health and social policy a number of parallel developments are reflected in the area of mental health. The Vagrancy Act of 1744 not only highlighted a continuing concern with vagrancy, but marked the differential treatment of 'lunatics' as opposed to vagrants which under the previous legislation, the Vagrancy Act of 1714, had been unclear, although the former were not to be subjected to whipping. The 1744 Act recommended the setting up of asylums for criminal and pauper lunatics with the decision for admission resting with Justices of the Peace rather than with physicians. This represents one of many legislative initiatives to deal with what was seen to be a growing problem of social order rather than a concern for legal rights.

The Vagrancy Act of 1744 stated that 'rogues, vagabonds and beggars' were to be incarcerated for up to one month in a local house of correction, and 'lunatics' or other mentally disordered people were to be maintained and cared for as long as was deemed necessary at the expense of local parishes. Such care was provided in the workhouse, small local hospitals or asylums, including private madhouses which until 1744 were not subject to any form of external monitoring, the latter having been described as an *'unregulated trade in lunacy'* (Murphy 1991: 29).

The 'madness' of King George III, although now understood as porphyria, a metabolic disorder, raised the profile and public interest in mental disorder alongside the introduction of ideas concerning the humane treatment and cure of insanity. In France, Philippe Pinel moved away from a regime based on confinement and custodial care to one where a firm but kind approach was supported by good physical care and a broadly therapeutic emphasis. Similar developments in Britain were implemented by, for example, William Tuke, a Quaker, who was responsible for the setting-up of the 'Retreat' in York in 1796 and introducing the notion of 'moral treatment'. Although such approaches did not become widespread, they contributed to a sense that treatment and cure were possible and, at one level, were influential in the groundswell towards increasing the number of asylums. Scull (1977) also suggests that the fact that moral treatment was not seen as the province of any particular professional group contributed to its limited development and application.

The presence of mentally disordered people within the workhouse population, however, remained problematic and, alongside the vision of the therapeutic care afforded by the new regimes of moral treatment, contributed the move towards the systematic establishment of county asylums. This was initiated by the County Asylums Act of 1808 and formally instituted by the 1845 Lunacy Act. This Act required the establishment of an asylum in every county in England and Wales.

In considering the design of the asylum buildings, it is interesting to note that whilst there was little obvious evidence of physical restraint in the form of barred windows, a feature of many of the asylum buildings was an emphasis on supervision. For example, 'crow's nests' were situated in stairwells which enabled the observation of all rooms and corridors and, in addition to the oversight of inmates, Samuel Tuke, the grandson of William, advocated the notion of 'espionage' which enabled the reciprocal supervision of senior and junior staff to ensure proper conduct. Arrangements such as these can be seen as examples of Foucault's concept of the 'panopticon' regarded as a means of ensuring total supervision and the internalization of the external gaze.

Throughout the nineteenth century there is evidence of the increasing salience of a biological model in understanding mental illness, supported by the discovery of the effective treatment of syphilis leading to the virtual elimination of 'paralysis of the insane'. Within physical medicine, the advances in understanding offered by the work of Koch and Pasteur which looked at the underlying causation of the disease process – notwithstanding the wider issues of the social environment which contributed to the causation and spread of disease – helped increase the acceptance of a biologically based medical model. Such developments also further promoted the notion that disease was outwith the control of any individual who could only look to the medical profession for a cure, and the allied conventions of patient passivity in the face of medical expertise.

Despite some changes, the asylums remained a key feature of mental health provision for virtually 100 years until the 1950s when numbers peaked and thereafter began to decline. As numbers of patients increased during the middle of the nineteenth century, the prevailing ethos was one of containment and custodianship and continuing use of physical treatments and restraint. Although nominally under the overall supervision of doctors, as the 1828 Asylum Act had specified that all asylums were required to have medical supervision, attendants offered a minimal level of care within a generally poor physical environment. Cure and discharge rates were low and almost matched by the numbers of people who died during their stay. The work of Darwin and others has also been seen to contribute to the notion of 'psychiatric Darwinism' which Treacher and Baruch (1980: 131) suggest legitimized the idea of incurability due to hereditary factors in the causation of disease.

Whilst there were some concerns as to the standard of care offered to patients, legislation enacted within the Lunacy Act of 1890 was primarily concerned with wrongful detention, rather than the fate of those who remained legally incarcerated. Rogers and Pilgrim (1996) refer to a 'symbiosis' of state (legislative and judicial) and medical interests as characterizing the era of the asylums and this relationship can continue to be traced well into the twentieth century. It is important to note, however, as pointed out by Campbell (1996), that there has always been a protest from people about the forms of treatment on offer. These include 'The Petition of the Poor Distracted People in the House of Bedlam' (1620) and attempts in the nineteenth century to counter the negative care in the asylums, such as the Alleged Lunatics' Friends Society formed in 1845 by John Perceval and others, with Perceval having written of his own experiences in the asylums.

Although the asylums provided a level of stability within the overall scene, other changes were taking place. The experiences of the First World War challenged previous notions of mental illness based upon genetic inferiority as soldiers and officers returned from the battlefield displaying symptoms of shock and stress. A recognition of environmental and social factors in the causation of mental distress, supported by a growing awareness of psychoanalysis and the publication of Freud's work, led to the establishment of the Tavistock Clinic. Child guidance clinics were also established, influenced by similar developments in the USA in the 1920s. These were based on the belief that timely intervention at an early stage could prevent later difficulties. The importance of attending to the needs of patients and their families was also recognized in the encouragement of the appointment of hospital almoners by the Royal Commission on Lunacy and Mental Disorder (1929) during this period. The 1930 Mental Treatment Act paved the way for voluntary admissions to asylums and recognized, although it did little to enforce, the need for outpatient clinics and psychiatry departments in general hospitals. Overall, this legislation is seen as strengthening the role of the medical profession over and above the legal/judicial aspects of care and treatment for those diagnosed as having mental illnesses and enabling the former to continue their role with the introduction of new treatments. Insulin therapy, psychosurgery and electro-convulsive therapy (ECT) were the new tools of the trade and by and large psychiatry continued to develop behind the closed doors of the asylums.

Preliminary discussions concerning the setting-up of the National Health Service (NHS) during and at the end of the Second World War largely overlooked the asylums, and it was only at a late stage in the process that they were included within mainstream provision and the purview of the regional hospital boards. The National Health Service Act (1946) also allocated responsibility to the local authorities for removal to hospital and the supervision and guardianship of 'mental defectives' in the community. This split between the health service and the local authority represents a continuing theme which will be examined later in this chapter as the development of community care has continued through the second half of the twentieth century to generate forceful exhortations for collaborative and joint working.

Many commentators have explored the rationale for the development of the welfare state, exemplified by the creation of the NHS. It has been seen as the culmination of a process which began with the First World War and was linked to continuing political concern with the overall health of the nation. This was associated with the need to maintain international political hegemony within the context of imperialism and to avoid social and political unrest at home. Underpinned by the earlier introduction of health insurance and pensions by the Liberal government from 1908, the vision of Beveridge was predicated on full employment for white males and the convention of a social wage with which a man could support his wife and children.

With regard to de-institutionalization, the numbers of beds occupied in the old asylums peaked in 1954 at 148,000 after which point there is a continuing decline in the figures, to 59,000 in 1990. The cause of this decline has been subject to considerable debate involving the increasing financial cost of institutional care, a growing concern regarding the negative effects of institutionalization and the introduction of new pharmacological treatments.

Although much has been written concerning the impact of new and apparently more effective medication, in particular the use of phenothyazines including chlorpromazine, anti-psychotic medication can only be seen as a contributory factor to a process which was already gathering momentum. The effectiveness of medication was clearly not uniformly distributed amongst the entire population of the asylums and although more beneficial results were noted in relation to acute rather than long-term illnesses, there were increasing concerns about side effects including tardive dyskinesia, or the involuntary shaking associated with prolonged use. It is also significant that the decline in institutional care was not confined to those diagnosed as mentally ill, but was also a factor in the care of other groups such as people with learning disabilities and older people where the use of 'new' medication was less widespread. Indeed many (Scull 1977; Treacher and Baruch 1980: 146) suggest that the so-called drug revolution had only partial significance in the wider changes taking place at this time.

Concerns about the use of medication within a primarily biological model of illness were also raised by the exponents of an increasingly critical view of psychiatry. One strand of this was fuelled by the work of Goffman (1961) whose critique of institutional care in all areas including hospital, residential schools and prisons highlighted the damage caused by total institutions based on impersonal, hierarchical and routine-ized care. This was subsequently supported by the evidence of hospital inquiries which drew attention to neglect, poor treatment and abuse in a number of settings. This was underpinned by the segregation of people diagnosed as having mental illness, physically demonstrated by the isolated location of many institutions and reinforced by the view that those diagnosed as having mental illnesses were undeserving of humane care and treatment.

The financial expense of maintaining costly institutions was also a factor in the process of decline which became increasingly pertinent as de-institutionalization continued. The 1959 Mental Health Act promoted the inclusion of mental health services within district general hospitals and there were many within psychiatry who welcomed the opportunity to move towards the mainstream of medical practice and the recognition it offered. The 1962 Hospital Plan launched by the then Health Minister Enoch Powell acting on an agenda of cutting expenditure on public services, promoted the closure of the old institutions described as antiquated and Victorian and their replacement by community services and the integration of psychiatric care within mainstream health care. However, little financial backing was forthcoming for the development of community facilities. As the movement towards the reintegration of patients into the community gathered momentum, the costs of maintaining large and complex hospital sites, demanding continuing staffing and maintenance, increased; a process made more costly by the loss of more able patients and the need to provide continuing care for those who were seen to be less likely candidates for rehabilitation.

COMMUNITY CARE – THE SECOND HALF OF THE TWENTIETH CENTURY

In reality whilst community care is regarded as a modern concept associated with social policy over the last twenty years, its origins can be seen in developments since 1948 and in the dismantling of the workhouse system which had provided little more than basic shelter for older and/or vulnerable people. Institutional services for people with mental health problems as well as those with learning disabilities and older people as we have seen also came under scrutiny and the gradual closure of long-stay hospitals serving a variety of groups can be traced from the 1960s onwards. Although progress was initially slow, the pace gathered momentum – fuelled by a number of scandals over abuse and neglect.

The notion of care *in* the community was also supplemented by the idea of care *by* the community in an attempt to reduce the growing expenditure by local authorities and to some extent health care services, and replace it with care provided by families, neighbours and local voluntary groups. Changes in the supplementary benefits system in 1980 also caused a massive rise in expenditure as regulations enabled residents in homes to reclaim the fees and the owners of private residential homes increased their rates to capitalize on this arrangement. Local authorities began to see that rather than increase their service provision, it would be economically beneficial to transfer their services to the private sector, whilst the NHS also looked increasingly to the private sector to resolve its discharge problems. The effects of these measures on the social security budget and public expenditure were profound and the costs increased from £10 million in 1979 to £500 million in the mid-1980s.

In 1986 the Audit Commission report (*Making a Reality of Community Care*) reviewed the fragmented range of services and criticized the variety of agencies involved and the often inappropriate care that was being provided. It also drew attention to the fact that more financial support was being directed towards hospital care than to local authorities who were trying to provide alternatives. In response to the short-fall in services for people leaving hospital, wide variations within and between geographical areas were identified. As a result of the paucity of joint working between local authorities and health authorities, the Audit Commission also drew attention to the potential deployment of a case management system, drawing on work in the USA and the development of alternatives to inpatient care for mental health services (Stein and Test 1980). A review of community care policy was commissioned with the particular brief:

> To review the way in which public funds are used to support community care policy and to advise the Secretary of State on options which would improve the use of these funds.
>
> (Griffiths 1988: 8)

The review was undertaken by Sir Roy Griffiths whose proposals were accepted and incorporated into the 1989 White Paper – *Caring for People* (Department of Health [DOH] 1989). The key objectives of the White Paper included the need to promote the development of domiciliary, day and respite care to enable people to live in their own homes; to provide support for carers; to make proper assessment of need and good case management the cornerstone of high-quality care; to promote a flourishing independent sector; to clarify the responsibilities of agencies, notably between the NHS and local authorities; and overall, to secure better value for taxpayers' money.

Additionally social services departments were charged with producing community care plans for their areas and for setting objectives, undertaking this task in consultation with local people and voluntary organizations. The resulting legislation in the form of the National Health Service and Community Care Act (1990) incorporated most of these objectives and emphasized the need for a purchaser/provider split and inter-agency collaboration, as well as introducing new systems of care management.

THE 'CRISIS' IN COMMUNITY CARE

Whilst a number of inquiries into the care of patients in long-stay hospitals (Martin 1985) had also provided a backdrop for community care reform, the move away from the provision of institutional care also brought its own crises. The killing of Isabel Schwartz, a social worker, by her former client, Sharon Campbell, in 1984, the actions of Michael Buchanan in 1992, who, following his discharge from hospital, killed a stranger (Frederick Gaver) in a car park and the stabbing of Jonathan Zito by Christopher Clunis, three months after discharge, in an unprovoked attack at a tube station, all raised wide and highly sensationalized concerns about the apparent dangers of supporting people in the community. In the early 1990s, events concerning Ben Silcock who entered the lions' enclosure at London Zoo and the death of Jonathan Newby, a 22-year-old volunteer care worker at a hostel in Oxford who was attacked and killed by John Rous, diagnosed with schizophrenia, also contributed to growing concern about safety. In 1993 Andrew Robinson attacked Georgina Robinson, an occupational therapist at the Edith Morgan Unit, South Devon, where he was a patient and further deaths included the stabbing of Bryan Bennet by Stephen Laudat in 1994 at a day centre in Newham and the killing by Kenneth Gray of his mother in 1995, after his transfer from a secure to an open ward.

Added to this catalogue of events should also be the deaths of those diagnosed as mentally ill which have themselves been attributed to the inadequacy or inappropriateness of services, such as Orville Blackwood at Broadmoor (1991), and the Committee of Enquiry's report which highlighted common factors involved in the deaths of two other African-Caribbean patients (HMSO 1992).

The findings of the Confidential Inquiry into Homicides and Suicides by Mentally Ill People reported in 1994 (Boyd 1994) that people in contact with mental health services prior to any attack were responsible for only 3% of homicides in a 12-month period. It was highlighted that only two victims in their study were randomly killed and none of the homicides had been committed by patients discharged from long-stay hospitals. They concluded that while the risk of homicide may be marginally higher for people suffering from mental health problems than for the population as a whole, the risk is actually very low. However, the heavily publicized deaths and the events surrounding them had created an atmosphere of anxiety and alarm which the findings did little to allay. In particular the killing of Jonathan Zito provided a touchstone for a sense of media-fuelled public panic which in turn led to a wide-ranging review of services. Reports pointed to a lack of specialist expertise, poor co-ordination of services, a failure to respond to warning signs and a lack of long-term accommodation for those with the most severe mental health problems. There were also concerns that 'race' was a factor in the limited care that Clunis received (Ritchie 1994).

A number of policy initiatives were introduced at this time which can be seen to relate directly to the widespread concern about risk. These included the Care Programme Approach in 1991, the introduction of supervision registers under Health Service Guidelines in 1994 and an amendment to the 1983 Mental Health Act in the form of the Mental Health (Patients in the Community) Act in 1995. These measures represented an attempt to ensure the co-ordinated delivery of services by introducing the Care Programme Approach and the identification of a key worker, by providing a means of targeting individuals who were the subject of particular concern regarding risk via the supervision registers (discontinued from 2001) and by bringing in a system of supervised discharge for patients detained under certain sections of the Mental Health Act (1983). The monitoring of risk and a concern to reassure the public that action was being taken clearly permeate each of these developments.

Overall, current mental health policy has to be located within the wider picture of health and social care and the development of a mixed economy of care, marked by the NHS and Community Care Act (1990). Many of the developments initiated by the Conservative government have remained in place since 1997 when the Labour government commenced its 'modernization' agenda. In respect of mental health, *Modernising Mental Health Services: Safe, Sound and Supportive* (DOH 1998) was regarded as providing a blueprint for continuing reform and innovation whilst emphasizing the need to reduce the risk which was seen to be associated with mental illness. This concern continues to influence policy and legislation and can be seen in the reform of the 1983 Mental Health Act. These areas are reviewed in more depth in Chapter 5.

CONCLUDING REMARKS

A review of the historical underpinnings of contemporary policy and practice highlights key themes which have an ongoing relevance. These include the continuing concern with risk and dangerousness and the persisting association between developments in the field of mental health and prevailing political, social and economic trends. There can also clearly be seen to be an enduring emphasis on the modernist tenets of science, progress and rationality and a concentration on mental distress as an illness with medical remedies. However, there are also indications of how dominant perspectives have been subject to resistance and challenge. In Chapter 5 the tension, paradox and inconsistency which can be seen to characterize current policy will be examined.

4 Inclusiveness and exclusiveness

Not only is the concept of illness different across cultures but also the ways in which illnesses are perceived.

(Fernando 2002: 40)

The concentration on biology in examining gender differences in the origins of mental disorder is over-determined . . . the tendency to 'naturalise' all gender differences, to see them as rooted in nature not culture, strengthens and confirms this biological orientation and, in contexts where women are typically subordinated, is frequently associated with assumptions of female biological inferiority.

(Busfield 1996: 165)

Given the current emphasis on social inclusion in government policy documents, an examination of inclusiveness and exclusiveness in current mental health policy and practice, with particular emphasis being paid to gender and ethnicity, becomes imperative. There has been much written about women and mental health, gender and mental health, and racism and mental health[1] and this chapter will explore the diverse ways in which gender and ethnicity have influenced understandings and how these have been translated into policy and practice. In this context, attention is paid to the over-representation of black and minority ethnic groups in the more controlling aspects of service provision and the under-representation of such groups in therapeutic support services. The greater likelihood of women receiving a diagnosis of 'depression' as opposed to men is also scrutinized.

With regard to differences associated with gender, ethnicity, class and sexuality, it is common practice to use statistics to demonstrate trends.

1 Key authors in relation to the former include Showalter (1987); Ussher (1991); Busfield (1996); Barnes and Maple (1992); Prior (1999). With regard to the latter area, those whose work has been influential include Bagley (1971); Cochrane (1977); Carpenter and Brockington (1980); McGovern and Cope (1987); Littlewood and Lipsedge (1981); Ineichen et al (1984); Fernando (1991; 1995; 2002); Rogers and Pilgrim (2003).

Class, for example, is seen to feature significantly as a possible determinant of mental ill-health and statistics show a high prevalence rate for the diagnosis of mental health problems, such as schizophrenia, depression and antisocial personality disorder amongst those from social classes V and VI (Rogers and Pilgrim 2003). African-Caribbean men and Irish men and women also feature significantly in the UK figures (Ramon 1996; Rogers and Pilgrim 2003). This information is useful and can influence policy and practice in a variety of ways. It can, for example, be used to draw attention to the part played by social and environmental factors in the causation of mental distress and it can be used to direct more resources towards the most vulnerable groupings. Alternatively, it can be used to indicate that those with the least overt power are more vulnerable to the application of diagnostic labelling. A key point to be made is that any data can be subject to a variety of interpretations. There are also clear dangers involved in viewing statistics as immutable hard facts. The collection of any data can be inadvertently influenced by unacknowledged assumptions, the ways in which particular questions are posed, how questions are understood and responded to and the number and representativeness of the respondents involved. In this chapter, the different ways in which information can be interpreted will be placed in perspective by looking at explanations of statistics and research findings relating to women and 'depression', lesbians and gay men, and ethnicity and 'psychoses'.

WOMEN AND 'DEPRESSION'

Mental Health Statistics for England (Government Statistical Service) for 2003–2004 indicate that of the 47,884 people receiving a primary diagnosis of mood disorder, women comprised 61%. Kaplan and Sadock (1995) in a review of community-based epidemiological surveys of mood disorders found women to be twice as likely as men to be experiencing depression. Evidence concerning the international prevalence of depression amongst women also refers to the fact that whilst rates of illness vary between countries, overall figures suggest that depression is twice as high in women as it is in men (Murray and Lopez 1996; WHO 2000). The eighth biennial report of the Mental Health Act Commission (2002) similarly emphasized that women are over-represented in the mental health system and are more likely to receive medication than men. As highlighted there are a number of explanations which can be put forward and these are appraised in this section.

One key interpretation is that more women decide to seek help than men. Dohrenwend and Dohrenwend (1977) were amongst the first to report differences in attitudes, expectations and norms between men and women, with women being more likely to admit distress, to view their distress in mental health terms, and to be more accepting of psychiatric treatment. This explanation can be used to suggest that it is not that more women suffer from depression than men, but that more women seek help and therefore feature in the statistics more than men.

Another explanation focuses on arguments associated with a 'Social Causation' interpretation (see Chapter 2) and relates to women being subject to greater stressors and as a result becoming more vulnerable to depression. Brown and Harris's (1978) famous study of the social origins of depression supports this view. Brown and Harris (1978) identified certain vulnerability factors which could make a woman more susceptible to depression (clinically defined) if also confronted with a further significant and negative life event (for example, bereavement, illness or divorce). These vulnerability factors were identified as: loss of mother before age 11 (and poor subsequent care, Brown et al 1986); absence of a confiding relationship with a partner; lack of employment full- or part-time outside the home; and the presence at home of three or more children under 14. They also found that the depressive episode was likely to be more severe if the woman had suffered previously from clinically defined depression and was aged over 50. Women who had low self-esteem were also found to be more likely to suffer from depressive episodes than those with high self-esteem. The relationship between the incidence of depression in women and the experience of stress was also emphasized by feminists in the 1980s (Oakely 1981; Orbach 1983). Barnes and Maple in 1992 focused on the mixed messages women receive about appropriate behaviour and highlighted the increased vulnerability of women to socially determined stressors. As a result mainstream thinking and policy directives can be seen to have increasingly foregrounded social causational factors such as the impact of gender based violence, socio economic disadvantage and negative life experiences on women and to have associated these with the production of humiliation and powerlessness. (Brown et al 1995: Fishbach and Herbert 1997; Kawachi and Kennedy 1999).

With regard to older women and depression and interpretations drawn from social causation approaches, few studies have specifically addressed gender issues. Those which have been carried out have associated depression with adversity or loss or threat of loss and the meanings that events related to these factors contain. However, Dover and McWilliam (1992) found in a study of 100 patients referred over a 30-month period to a psychogeriatric service with depression, that only 3% of the male inpatients and 29% of the female patients were physically well. In line with this finding they found many drug treatments for serious illnesses are known either to cause or to increase a depressive mood.

Another way of looking at how more women come to feature more prominently in mental health statistics relating to depression than men draws from social constructionist perspectives. A question that can be posed is: 'Are problems reported to GPs more likely to be interpreted/constructed as mental health problems than those reported by men?'. Broverman et al in 1970 famously highlighted that many clinicians viewed a typically healthy adult in terms of stereotypical and idealized male characteristics. This placed women in a 'no win' situation. If a woman conformed to the stereotypical idealized view of womanhood, she was found not to be mentally healthy although she could be regarded as a 'normal' woman. If she deviated, she was found not only to be mentally unhealthy, but potentially in need of control. Research by Goldberg and Huxley in 1980, indicated that GPs defined more women as suffering from mental health difficulties than men. Similarly Cochrane in 1983 drew attention to findings which showed more women than men being referred for specialist psychiatric help. There is also evidence tht women are more likely than men to be prescribed psychotropic medication (Gorman 1992; Simoni-Wasila 2000).

In the 1970s and 1980s, the analyses of 'second wave' feminists gave particular impetus to social constructionist perspectives (for example, Chesler 1972; Showalter 1987; Ussher 1991). Ussher commented:

> For behaviour which is deemed in need of control, men will be more likely to go to prison and women to hospital, or to a regional secure unit . . . . With good behaviour, parole is automatic after two thirds of a prison sentence, but not at any time during a compulsory psychiatric detention. The implications of this are serious as women will be invariably confined for longer, and as many would argue that the stigma of a psychiatric detention is greater than that of a prison detention, the implication for women of this differential setting could be more long lasting.
>
> (Ussher 1991: 172)

More recently Busfield (1996) has drawn attention to the complex interaction of social constructionist and social causational influences. She states:

> Highlighting the importance of power to the analysis of gender and mental disorder points to the links between the denial of agency (power) that is often involved in judgements of mental disorder and the importance of powerlessness in understanding gender differences in the genesis of mental disorder. Women's relative lack of power in many situations in comparison with men, and the perceptions surrounding their lack of power, means they are doubly disadvantaged. On the one hand, their lack of power makes it more likely that their behaviours may be viewed as indicative of mental disorder. And, on the other hand, it makes certain experiences more traumatic or distressing. We cannot, however, make broad generalizations about which of these processes is more important where women are over-represented in patient populations since their relative importance will vary across time and place. Nor should we forget the regulation of male as well as female behaviour

both through definitions of mental disorder and by a variety of other means.

(Busfield 1996: 236–7)

Prior (1999) points to the way in which gendered language has changed in psychiatric texts over the last thirty years from gendered derogatory language to one which adopts a gender neutral approach. This she sees as being as a result of the influence of feminist and gay liberation movements. In order to explain why the accounts of 'survivors' continue to highlight how stereotypical assumptions about normal male and female behaviour influence diagnoses, she points to the ways in which changes in the academic literature are perhaps two decades ahead of current psychiatric practice.

Arguments drawing from social causation orientations and those informed by feminist analyses which adopt a more social constructionist perspective can be seen to have been influential, with, as has been mentioned, a social causation approach being most privileged in policy terms. This can be seen in MIND Policy papers (e.g. Gorman 1992) and the DOH consultation document *Women's Mental Health: Into the Mainstream: Strategic Development of Mental Health Care for Women* (2002a). However, although the impact of differential power relations and the effect of these on problem identification and response is insufficiently explored, increasingly emphasis is being placed on the need to incorporate women's concerns and experiences. This is particularly the case with regard to recognizing the impact of violence and sexual abuse on women and the importance of women-only psychiatric wards. However, although *The NHS Plan* (DOH 2000b) specifically refers to the development of day services for women, the safety of women on mixed-sex wards and the adequacy of appropriate child care provision for those responsible for children, the picture overall remains mixed. Change has taken place, although, at a wider level, the emphasis on risk and dangerousness can be viewed as shifting attention away from women's mental health needs to those of men who are constructed as psychotic and dangerous.

LESBIANS AND GAY MEN

The mental health of lesbians and gay men also merits attention, not least due to the historical identification of homosexuality as a mental illness, only declassified in the Diagnostic and Statistical Manual of Mental Disorders (DSM) in 1973 and remaining in the *International Statistical Classification of Diseases and Related Health Problems* (ICD) until 1992 (see WHO 1990). As a diagnosable condition, homosexuality was 'treated' with a range of dubious and ill-founded interventions including aversion therapy and electric shock treatment until late in the twentieth century. Paradoxically, one consequence of increasing the visibility of various lifestyle choices and sexual behaviours, has been the exchange of a diagnostic process whereby to be attracted to the same sex was in and of itself an illness, to, in the experience of many lesbians and gay men, an assumption that mental health difficulties must be rooted in sexuality to the exclusion of any other issues and experiences.

As with issues of 'race' and gender, once again perspectives drawing on both social construction and social causation arguments contribute to our understanding and, in reality, are interrelated. With regard to the former, notions of normality and abnormality in relation to sexual desire and behaviour, associated with the development of the disciplines of psychiatry and psychology and coupled with existing moral disapproval, together created and maintained the historical conditions within which homophobia could flourish. This in turn fuelled the stigma and prejudice experienced by many lesbians and gay men who found themselves at best social outcasts and at worst victims of physical violence, whilst at the same time being denied equality in terms of legislative protection with regard to access to housing, employment, pensions, as well as discrimination concerning family life and relationships. A 1998 survey in England of 4,000 lesbians and gay men found that 34% of men and 24% of women had experienced violence because of their sexuality, 32% had been harassed in the last five years and 73% had been called names. Bullying has also been found to be severe in schools (Rivers 1995).

It is perhaps not surprising that, in the absence of other supporting or protective factors, many lesbians and gay men may experience the breakdown of family relationships and/or the need to assume a pretended heterosexuality, with severe consequences for self-esteem and the internalization of oppression. Rivers found that of 190 lesbian and gay young people surveyed, over half had contemplated self-harm and 40% had attempted suicide at least once. Other researchers refer to an increased risk of suicide and self-harm (Bridget and Lucille 1996; Faulkner and Cranston 1998).

In terms of accessing mental health services Golding (1997) found that lesbians, gay men and bisexuals may not feel able to disclose their identity with 78% expressing reservations about whether it was safe enough to do so and 84% fearing prejudice or being pathologized. Additionally, many participants experienced ignorance, stereotyping, voyeurism, judgemental attitudes and the trivialization of relationships. Continuing prejudice also continues to affect the training opportunities for therapists and there is a continuing resistance to self-disclosure amongst gay and lesbian mental health professionals, in effect, maintaining silence and the presumption of heterosexuality (Bartlett et al 2001).

King and McKeown (2003) found that lesbians, gay men and bisexual people are at greater risk of psychological problems including substance misuse and that gay men and lesbians were more likely to consult their GP for emotional difficulties. Whilst many did not report outright rejection in their dealings with mental health professionals there was a level of concern regarding inappropriate responses and a strong recommendation made for training for workers to ensure understanding and sensitivity.

'RACE' AND ETHNICITY

When looking at 'race', ethnicity and 'psychosis', both the statistics and the research findings can be seen to present a particular picture and one which is by now fairly well known. Bagley (1971) and Cochrane (1977) drew attention in the 1970s to the diagnosis of schizophrenia being given more frequently to people from immigrant groups in Britain than those born in the UK. Carpenter and Brockington's 1980 study in Manchester and Dean et al's 1981 study in south-east England found this was particularly the case for people originating in Africa, Asia and the Caribbean. Littlewood and Lipsedge in 1981 emphasised the misdiagnosis of schizophrenia among black patients and McGovern and Cope in 1987 surveyed patients compulsorily detained in a hospital in Birmingham and found that approximately two thirds of black patients, compared to one third of white patients, were diagnosed as suffering from schizophrenia. Sashidharan (1993) found that in some African-Caribbean communities the incidence of schizophrenia was ten times higher than would usually be expected. Lloyd and Moodley in 1992 examined the psychiatric inpatient population in the catchment area of the Bethlem and Maudsley Hospitals. They found more African-Caribbean than white people being given anti-psychotic medication and discovered that this was because a larger proportion of black patients had been given a diagnosis of schizophrenia. Overall they found that black patients were significantly more likely to be receiving depot anti-psychotic medication, to be detained under a section of the Mental Health Act, and to have been involved in a violent incident during admission.

Ineichen et al in 1984 and Ineichen in 1990; McGovern and Cope in 1987; Harrison et al in 1984 and 1989; Barnes, Bowl and Fisher in 1990; and Bean et al in 1991: all have shown black patients being over-represented among compulsorily detained patients in hospital. Similarly, Littlewood and Cross (1980), Shaikh (1985) and Rogers and Pilgrim (1996) have pointed to the apparent overuse of ECT in the treatment of African-Caribbean and Asian patients. Persaud (1993–4), when looking at demographic factors, highlighted that, if the number of African-Caribbean people in the population by using head of household statistics from earlier census data is underestimated, there will automatically be an overestimation of the rate of illness in the population. However, the over-representation of African-Caribbean men in the statistics for schizophrenia and amongst those compulsorily detained in hospital is now generally accepted and the need for government action has been highlighted (e.g. *Inside/Outside*, DOH 2003c).

Across Europe, the picture is mixed. In France, North Africans have a higher rate of identified mental distress than Africans generally, whilst throughout Europe, including the UK, men and women from the Indian subcontinent are recorded as having a lower than average incidence. Reasons given include generally higher socio-economic status, a reluctance to engage with Eurocentric services and the use of alternative healers within communities (Ramon 1996). As highlighted in the Introduction, Irish people in both Britain and Ireland also feature significantly in the statistics, with emphasis being placed on possible causative factors such as the ongoing effects of oppression and colonialism and the fact that in Britain, many Irish people fall into lower socio-economic groups (Rogers and Pilgrim 2003).

When looking at explanations for the higher incidence of African-Caribbean men being subject to compulsory detention, as with the discussions surrounding 'women and depression', conflicting views have been put forward. The 'Increased Stressors' explanation focuses on poverty, unemployment and racism all contributing to placing increased stress upon certain communities which in turn increases the risk of mental ill-health (e.g. Cope 1989). Fanon (1967) focused on how life within a colonial system influences the personalities of those colonized. Being treated as intellectually and morally inferior in an individual's own country can lead to an internalization of inferiority and ambiguity and anger directed at the self as well as at the colonizer. The 'Increased Stressor' argument can be associated with social causation approaches (see Chapter 2). However, the following 'Social Control' and 'Racist' arguments can be clearly linked to social constructionist orientations.

The 'Social Control' approach looks at the over-representation of black people in psychiatric statistics as an indication of the way that psychiatry forms part of the social control apparatus which focuses particularly on black people. Francis (1988), for example, sees the criminalization and medicalization of black people as a connected process. The 'Racist' argument highlights racism within psychiatric theory and practice. Suman Fernando in 1991 asserted: '. . . racism in psychiatry is not an aberration – it is the normal condition, and secondly, it is not the recognition of cultural differences that is racist, but the attribution of values to these differences' (1991: 115). Littlewood in 1992 maintained that understanding psychiatric problems among Britain's black and minority ethnic population has to take racism into account. Fernando, Ndegwa and Wilson (1998) in turn argued that forensic psychiatric services are not appropriately serving multi-ethnic societies because of the ways in which 'race', schizophrenia and criminality have historically been linked in Western Europe and the USA.

The issue of culture in relation to a discussion of 'race', ethnicity and mental health is an important one. Psychiatry, as it is currently practised, has developed and been informed by Western cultural beliefs and practices. In the 1980s the recognition of cultural differences led to the development of transcultural psychiatry. This approach continued to regard psychiatric diagnoses as objective and universal but drew attention to the ways in which cultural factors and language problems could affect how mental illnesses were presented, resulting in misunderstandings and misdiagnoses. This approach has been criticized for not taking account of the effects of racism. The extent to which an apartheid system could be maintained by the provision of separate services for black communities, building on the precepts of transcultural psychiatry, has also been highlighted (Bhui and Sashidharan 2003).

Yet another perspective focuses on rights and entitlements. When looking at issues of self-harm as they affect Asian women, notions of both cultural pathology and the dichotomous treatment of 'gender' and 'race' are challenged. The impact of abuse and violence is considered as a factor implicated in the mental health of women across all ethnic groups (Heise et al 1994) and explicitly identified with regard to Asian women, along with other social and economic pressures including racism and bullying, poverty, homelessness and family pressure (Chantler et al 2001; Newham Inner City Multifund and Newham Asian Women's Project 1998). Additionally, other evidence continues to suggest that Asian women may be especially prone to experience social conflict which includes dealing with changes in family expectations around social behaviour (Bhugra et al 1999).

In terms of access to services, there is also evidence that, prior to a crisis point being reached, many Asian women in particular are not aware of the range of services that might be available (Chantler et al 2001; Newham Inner City Multifund and Newham Asian Women's Project 1998). The question of the provision of, and access to, appropriate services, draws attention to the discriminatory processes which may shape and determine the pathways to obtaining support and, in turn, help-seeking behaviour. Such an analysis draws attention to the continuation of an underpinning discourse which looks to cultural explanations and hence changing individual and cultural beliefs rather than addressing fundamental inequalities in service provision. As an alternative, women seek the support of services they regard as being sensitive to their needs including refuges and specialist South Asian projects as well as some statutory sector services. Whilst these may be appropriate at one level, there is elsewhere, however, the suggestion, that women find themselves in a cycle of referrals between services, frequently within the voluntary sector, which are sensitive to culture and language and those, primarily in the statutory sector, namely health and social services, which offer sensitive and specifically directed mental health support (Green et al 2002). The resulting picture raises important issues of entitlement allied to fundamental notions of citizenship and inclusion as Asian women experiencing distress are effectively denied access to mainstream services and support.

The situation with regard to black and minority ethnic elders has also received relatively little attention. The Centre for Policy on Ageing (1998) undertook research looking at the information provided by statutory services to those black and minority ethnic elders experiencing mental health problems. The research concluded that 'absence, inaccuracy and inappropriateness tended to characterise the information provision for older people from black and minority ethnic groups' (1998: 11). Recommendations drawn from the research project included the importance of professionals getting to know the local population in terms of the diversity of cultures, histories and meanings beyond the census figures and statistical surveys. The importance of involving local people in the preparation and piloting of information provision was also highlighted as was the need to produce information materials in a variety of formats as a matter of course and to disseminate information beyond service locations to where older people live their day-to-day lives, following this up with personal contact as appropriate. The need for sufficient, well-utilized interpreting and other support services was also emphasized, together with the importance of updating information in line with changes in services and shifts in communities. Most importantly the need to look at issues of citizenship, participation and organizational imperatives was given priority.

Currently, as Fernando (2002) and Rogers and Pilgrim (2003) point out, psychiatry as a discipline has acknowledged both the operation of culturally specific disorders and those which are seen to have a universal relevance. This creates a clear tension. Rogers and Pilgrim (2003) state:

> Any substantial professional concession to the importance of 'emic' (culturally specific) disorders threatens to undermine psychiatry as a universally applicable form of medical science, but to deny their existence immediately invites accusations of Western intellectual imperialism or racism.
>
> (Rogers and Pilgrim 2003: 10)

Fernando (2002) highlights the contradiction between Western diagnoses of depression with antidepressants manufactured by Western drug firms being promoted in Africa and the marketing of Indian mysticism in North America. With regard to the acknowledgement of 'racism' and the importance of different cultural understandings of mental health, Fernando (2002) reports that the picture from within psychiatry remains bleak. However, he maintains that optimism can be drawn from the challenges to psychiatry and psychology from service user groups, voluntary organizations, major reports such as the MacPherson Report (1999) and the willingness of black and Asian people, including professionals and academics, to speak out against racism and to develop innovative, culturally sensitive approaches. However, it is also no surprise that many black people are wary of psychiatric services and fear differential treatment. Errol Francis (2003), a black mental health campaigner, says that many black people admitted to hospital believe they may die as a result of their contact with mental health services. 'Patients' and relatives also fear being subject to experiments. He says relatives 'see their loved one dribbling and suffering from gross side-effects and see other patients who don't appear to be so drugged up and they conclude that the only reason for this is some kind of experiment' (Francis 2003: 30). The death of David Bennett, originally diagnosed with drug-induced psychosis, further confirms such suspicions, as the inquiry (2003) found that he experienced racial abuse in hospital from patients and obtained limited community care.

As discussed in Chapter 2, 'madness' can be viewed as essentially 'other' with 'others' being identified as those who do not fit and who are seen as a potential threat. Pilgrim and Rogers (1999) link the concept of 'otherness' to a form of racism which is concerned with mechanisms of inclusion and exclusion associated with the legacy of ex-colonized and ex-colonizer. Racism is about the fixing of difference. The association of black men with mental illness compounds this fixing of difference and gives it a legitimizing medicalized twist.

A further illustration of this may be found if the situation of Irish people in Britain is considered in more detail. As a white minority ethnic group, Irish-born people make up 1.5% of the British population, rising to 4.6% if those with Irish-born parents are included, and form the largest migrant minority in Western Europe, totalling 2.5 million. Irish men have been found to be the only migrant group to experience worsening of life expectancy on migration with the social class profile of Irish people being closest to that of the African-Caribbean population. Consequently, Irish people are more likely to sleep rough in London than black people or Asian people, are more likely to suffer discrimination in the criminal justice system and are clearly over-represented in mental health services. However, mental health issues within the Irish community are frequently characterized as invisible and undifferentiated from the white British majority. A recent report from the Department of Health (April 2004) also highlights dissatisfaction from Irish people (94%) as being more likely than that expressed by black people (88%), Asian people (86%) or Chinese people (44%) in terms of seeing staff cultural awareness as a problem. Nearly half reported negative experiences citing racial discrimination linked to cultural insecurity, stereotyping and exclusion.

With regard to the construction of black men as violent, Taylor (2004) looks at how this has resulted in both a preponderance of pharmaceutical control and a reluctance to explore this issue in greater depth. He recognizes how the process of being constructed as 'other' carries with it the attribution of negative characteristics such as violence, lack of control and lack of insight, but explores the ways in which anger and rage have been incorporated into understandings of black masculinity by black men themselves. He points to the work of Marriott (2000) who, building on the analysis of Fanon, maintains that 'anger has long been a chosen vocation for black men desperate to retain their separateness' (Marriott 2000: viii–ix). Similarly, he draws attention to the work of Hooks (1995) who argues that work in the field of mental health needs to combine emotional healing with politicization and social activism. She focuses on the importance of understanding rage as a potential healing response to oppression and exploitation. Taylor (2004) juxtaposes Hooks's observation on the media representation of black rage as useless, meaningless and destructive with her insights into the therapeutic potential of rage. He recognizes the calls of black feminists not to use social conditions to exonerate the sexism and exploitation shown by some black men towards black women but uses the circumstances surrounding the fatal stabbing of Jonathan Zito by Christopher Clunis in 1992 to argue for a more nuanced analytical approach to unravelling taken-for-granted explanations. In relation to media-fuelled public anxiety, this event has come to epitomize the danger posed by 'untreated schizophrenics' to unrelated members of the public as Christopher Clunis, a black man with a diagnosis of schizophrenia, fatally stabbed a passenger, Jonathan Zito, unknown to him, at Finsbury Park tube station in 1992. As discussed, this event fuelled a range of measures including risk assessment, assertive outreach and compulsory treatment in the community. It is also often portrayed as having resulted from the failure of a range of agencies to ensure that Clunis took the high doses of neuroleptic medication prescribed. The fact that Clunis is black was also seen to encourage some agencies not to assertively engage with and treat Clunis fearing charges of racism (Ritchie Inquiry 1994). Taylor (2004) focuses on less publicized information such as Clunis's attempt to renegotiate the high levels of chlorpromazine he was prescribed and the lack of support he received following the death of a girlfriend and his mother. He criticizes the complacency and acquiescence of the inquiry in relation to a total drugs policy and the failure to recognize the feelings of rage so commonly associated with grief and loss.

The killing of Jonathan Zito was undeniably tragic, but the dominant interpretation and solution inflexibly deny other understandings and responses. This is not only unhelpful to those experiencing distress, but can be counterproductive with regard to current policy directives. If the only available response is compulsory treatment, then, like Clunis, those in distress can unilaterally withdraw from taking all medication and avoid contact with mental health professionals. Assertive outreach and controlling solutions faced with non-compliant individuals can have only limited effect.

This discussion leads on to a further exploration of current interpretations of risk and dangerousness. (This area is also appraised in Chapters 3 and 5.) These two terms have been combined so frequently, that the linkage has become firmly established in the minds of many. Debates about risk can be broadly linked to Beck's seminal work on the risk society published in 1992. Beck (1992) associated 'risk' with the ways in which society deals with the dangers brought about by post-industrial modernization. He particularly emphasized the political and social dynamics of risk arguing that due to the processes of globalization and modernization, the risks experienced today are very different to those experienced previously. Accordingly, what was previously considered safe, now carries with it elements of risk. Douglas and Wildavsky (1982) pointed to the influence of social and cultural factors in determining those risks chosen for individual and societal attention. They contended that societies selectively choose certain risks for attention and that 'risk' has to be conceptualized as a social process rather than as an objective reality. With regard to mental health, the ways in which the concept of risk has become associated with harm or danger have resulted in the assumption that there is a direct correlation and that risk can be scientifically and objectively calculated. Alaszewski (1998) emphasized the positive aspects of risk-taking and this is clearly an aspect of 'risk' often overlooked. The uncoupling of risk and dangerousness is necessary to appreciate that both have very different meanings and implications. Risk is primarily about uncertainty and weighing up the balance of positive or negative outcomes. Danger, on the other hand, refers to a specific state. Assessments focusing on the risk of dangerousness are, by their very nature, subjective. There are areas which have been highlighted as being linked to an increased risk of violence to others for those who have had previous contact with mental health services. These include a history of violent behaviour, more complex treatment needs, alcohol or drug misuse, medication non compliance and a loss of contact with services (National Confidential Inquiry into Suicide and Homicide by People with Mental Illness 2001). However, as pointed out by Parton (1998), the implications of calculability and objectivity inherent to the risk concept are problematic. 'Risk' is inherently contingent and open to differing and sometimes conflicting interpretation. According to Shaw and Shaw (2001), a greater focus on notions of uncertainty and ambiguity is called for in social welfare work, where much experience is not characterized by scientific calculations of risk, but imbued with intuition and uncertainty.

Langan (1999) draws attention to how an individualized perspective on risk factors fails to take account of the complex contextual nature of risk as it is shaped by social, economic and political factors. J Smith (2001) takes this further and maintains in relation to social work that social workers' central concern with the assessment and management of risk, in relation to vulnerable people, cannot be sustained. He calls for social workers to 'abandon the spurious expectation that they can predict conditions and outcomes of risk'. He calls for a focus on 'uncertainty and ambiguity' and for the potential creativity that this unleashes to be exploited (2001: 289–90).

PRESSURE FOR ACTION

Government documents such as *Inside/Outside* (DOH 2003c) have acknowledged the need for action with regard to racism both in relation to official bodies and statutory services 'inside', and the voluntary sector and black and minority ethnic communities 'outside'. This report accepts that institutionalized racism exists within mental health services, that there is an overemphasis on institutional and coercive models of care, and that priority is given to institutional needs over individual needs and rights. It stresses the importance of including ethnic inequalities in relation to the standards incorporated within the *National Service Framework for Mental Health* (DOH 1999a) and emphasizes the professional skills required for practice in a multicultural society with pointers being given for professional training.

Inside/Outside (DOH 2003c) has clearly informed the DOH's draft document *Delivering Race Equality: A Framework for Action* (2003a). However, views are divided on the message being delivered by the DOH and the action being proposed. Louis Appleby, the mental health 'tsar' in post when the 2003 draft was published, maintained that changes could best be achieved by means of star ratings and inspections by the Commission for Health Improvement rather than by setting out a strategy with clear targets. He accepted that 'institutional racism', defined as meaning that mental health services do not 'operate equally to the benefit of all ethnic groups, so some people are disadvantaged by the way the system works', does exist and acknowledged that services need to be 'less conventional' (Leason 2003: 18–19). He also recommended the inclusion of ethnicity in assessment criteria and the development of a performance indicator specifically related to ethnicity as well as mandatory minority ethnic representation on trust boards. However, Sashidharan, a member of the External Reference Group for *Inside/Outside*, believes that the DOH document diluted the major recommendations of *Inside/Outside*. Sashidharan is quoted as saying: 'The experience of working with the DOH around this document and subsequently, has reinforced my view that this is an example of institutionally racist attitudes and behaviours on its part' (Sashidharan 2003: 18).

Fernando (2003) maintains that action is urgently needed in a number of related areas. His list of areas to be prioritized includes the following:

- changing professional training in order to address its Eurocentric nature and embedded racist attitudes;
- remodelling the process of mental health assessment in order to incorporate Asian and African worldviews and psychology, especially spirituality;
- diminishing the power accorded to the diagnostic system, especially that of 'schizophrenia';
- minimizing institutional racism in service provision;
- altering the power structure within the mental health workforce;
- countering discrimination in the employment of staff;
- reducing racism in sectioning procedures, especially in the forensic field;
- incorporating an anti-racist element in risk assessment;
- strengthening the funding and organization of the black voluntary sector.

Like Sashidharan, Fernando advocates the setting of targets with clearly identified practical strategies. He states: 'We know from past experience that general good intentions (as propounded in past dialogue documents) do not get translated into actual changes' (Fernando 2003: 22).

CONCLUDING REMARKS

It is important to acknowledge that differences associated with gender and ethnicity do not operate in isolation but intersect and interact with other differences such as class and sexuality. Historical location and cultural location have also to be seen as major influencing factors together with the specific contexts in which forms of interaction take place. Many authors (for example, Prior 1999; Rogers and Pilgrim 1999; and Fernando 2002) have drawn attention, not only to the influence of gender and racialized stereotypes, but also to the ways in which psychiatrists have been caricatured as social control agents, misogynists and racists. Rogers and Pilgrim (1999) see part of the problem resulting from the divergence between sociology and psychiatry over the past thirty years. Whilst psychiatry has focused increasingly on improving the reliability and validity of diagnostic constructs (for example, the American Psychiatric Association's DSM III and DSM IV, sociologists have tended to look at mental illness as a social construct with associated 'stigmatising, coercive and ideological intent' (Rogers and Pilgrim 1999: 43). In this context they prioritize a social causation approach and argue that both psychiatry and sociology have paid insufficient attention to causal explanations and frameworks relating to the inverse relationship between mental health and social position. The argument put forward in this chapter is that social constructionist as well as social causationist perspectives are productive but in context-specific situations there are clearly points when difference is translated into division, discrimination and oppression and that the issues raised have to inform debates about fostering inclusiveness within the very broad arena of mental health.

5 Contemporary policy: tension, paradox and inconsistency

> If we know what the problems are, why haven't we been able to develop successful solutions?
>
> ('Introduction, Cases for Change',
> National Institute for Mental Health in England [NIMHE] 2003b: 7)

This chapter explores current policy developments in relation to mental health in England and Wales. It takes account of similarities with the previous Conservative administration and the range of policies formulated since 1997. It further highlights the tension, paradox and inconsistency that these policies have produced and uses these as a means of constructively appraising key areas.

CURRENT POLICY

The final years of the twentieth and the beginning of the twenty-first century in Britain have seen a renewed interest in health and social care policy with a particular emphasis being placed on mental health. The incoming Labour government of 1997 has been responsible for the introduction of the 'modernization' agenda which focuses on improving the delivery and quality of services by drawing from an approach famously entitled the 'third way'. This sets out to avoid the excesses of either the Conservatives' concern with privatization or 'Old Labour's' preoccupation with the public ownership of services. However, although the Labour government, in its energetic takeover of power, appears ostensibly to have moved away from the policies associated with the previous Conservative administration and the legacy of 'Thatcherism',[1] in practice, the project of New Labour demonstrates a

---

1 Margaret Thatcher's time in office was characterized by attempts to 'roll back the frontiers of the state' by bringing market principles into welfare systems, by prioritizing private over public services, by emphasizing individual and family responsibility and by decreasing public spending on welfare.

marked level of continuity with policies hitherto associated with the Conservatives. This continuity includes an ongoing emphasis on family values, albeit in the context of diverse family forms, concerns with performance management and quantitatively orientated targets, the promotion of independence via welfare-to-work policies, and increasing public/private partnerships and finance arrangements. In relation to the latter, although the previous Conservative administration focused on establishing an internal market and a mixed economy of care (rather than the development of joint health and social care trusts, primary care trusts and the use of private capital to support the NHS), concerns with economy and efficiency, expressed as 'Best Value', continues to prevail. As with the Conservatives, New Labour's policies have also been set against a backdrop of economic and demographic pressures, vulnerability to the global economy and an ageing population (Fawcett, Featherstone and Goddard 2004).

New Labour's keynote policy document for mental health services was introduced in 1998 and entitled *Modernising Mental Health Services* (DOH 1998). In this document, particular importance was attached to providing comprehensive services and addressing gaps, especially in relation to those diagnosed with severe mental illnesses. Other provisions include increasing the number of inpatient beds and expanding assertive outreach and crisis teams. This emphasis can be seen to demonstrate the government's ongoing concern with safety and risk identification. There has also been a focus on clearly managed intervention strategies and systematic progress monitoring. *Modernising Mental Health Services* (1998) also set in motion the reform of the 1983 Mental Health Act which controversially included broadening the definition of mental disorder, the criteria for compulsion, and the use of community treatment orders.[2]

The *National Service Framework for Mental Health*, published in 1999 (DOH 1999a), is one of a number of frameworks for improving health and social care by the introduction of service performance monitoring mechanisms in seven key areas. Standard one focuses on mental health promotion, standards two and three on primary care and access to services, standards four and five on effective services for people with severe mental illness, standard six on caring about carers, and standard seven on preventing suicide. The *National Service Framework for Mental Health* also demonstrates the government's emphasis on clinical governance and evidence-based practice. It sets out a clear hierarchy of evidence with type one, regarded as the most important, incorporating systematic review with at least one randomized controlled trial and type five, viewed as the least important, referring to expert opinion, which includes the opinion of service users and carers. In association with the *National Service Framework*, the

2 The reform of the 1983 Mental Health Act additionally included replacing the role of approved social workers with approved mental health professionals and replacing the nearest relative with a 'nominated person' to look after the patient's interests.

revision of the Care Programme Approach, further draws attention to the government's concern with the management principle of 'getting people to the right place for the right intervention at the right time' (DOH 1999b).

The NHS Plan was introduced in 2000 and detailed changes to occur over the course of the next ten years. In line with the emphasis placed on the meeting of targets, it incorporates aspects such as the provision of 1,000 new graduate mental health staff to work in primary care, an extra 500 community mental health team workers, 50 early intervention teams to provide treatment and support to young people with psychosis, 335 crisis resolution teams, an increase to 220 assertive outreach teams, women-only day services, 700 extra staff to work with carers and more suitable accommodation for up to 400 people currently in high-secure hospitals (DOH 2000b; NIMHE 2003a). These proposals reflect the government's concerns regarding early intervention and the importance currently attached to reaching those not normally in contact with psychiatric services. There is also an emphasis on increasing support services, particularly for women, and as highlighted by the reform of the 1983 Mental Health Act, the further development of non-hospital-based forms of systematic intervention and follow-up.

Since 1997, the government has promulgated the concept of 'joined-up' thinking as a way of linking together key initiatives in a range of areas. New Labour's policy programme has emphasized joint planning and commissioning in the delivery of services and in the meeting of specified targets and outcomes. Programmes in the mental health arena have also been related to the wider agenda which focuses on tackling poverty, unemployment and social exclusion predominantly by means of 'welfare-to-work' policies. This approach underpins a range of current policy initiatives including the work of the Connexions service for young people and the Sure Start scheme for families and single parents with children under the age of 4. The Disability Discrimination Act (1995) has also strengthened the position of those assessed as disabled, by means of a 'chronic and enduring mental health problem', with regard to employment, access, goods and services.

The social inclusion platform adopted by New Labour has resulted in certain sections of the community receiving specific attention. The MacPherson Report (1999), for example, drew attention to ongoing racism in public services and the over-representation of some black and minority ethnic groups in areas of mental health services where there is an emphasis on compulsion. As seen in Chapter 4, there is controversy about the way forward, but government policy documents – for example, Inside/Outside (DOH 2003c); and Delivering Race Equality: A Framework for Action (DOH 2003a), demonstrate that attention is being paid to this area. Similarly, as highlighted above, the mental health needs of women have also been reviewed. In this respect, there has been an emphasis on the social causation of mental health difficulties with an explicit acknowledgement that issues of domestic violence and abuse, poverty, the experience of parenthood and other caring responsibilities take their toll on mental health. The needs of black and minority ethnic women, lesbians and older women are also starting to be recognized. At a practice level there are now requirements for single-sex wards and women-only facilities as part of an integrated approach to ensure gender-sensitive services throughout specialist mental health and primary care services (DOH 2002a; DOH 2003b).

The government has also paid attention to user involvement. The NHS Reform and Health Care Professionals Act (2002) has built on the statutory duty contained in the Health and Social Care Act (2001) for the NHS to involve and consult the public when planning or changing services. It is also now a statutory requirement for all trusts to establish patient forums and an independent complaints advisory service. A commission focusing on patient and public involvement in health has also been established.

At this stage, it is also useful to place the policy developments that are taking place in England and Wales in a broader context. This is a complex undertaking as, given the controversies that reign in this field with regard to definitions and responses, it is difficult to compare like with like. However, in relation to compulsory detention in hospital for observation and/or treatment, arguably the most contentious area, a recent study by Salize and Dressing (2004), focusing on the European Union (EU), has produced some interesting findings. Despite problems with the reliability and validity of data, clear differences can be observed in the compulsory admission rates per 100,000 of the population across Europe. Finland has the highest rate with 218 compulsory admissions, followed by Austria and Germany (175), Sweden (114), the UK and Luxembourg (93), Ireland (74), Belgium (47), the Netherlands (44), Denmark (34), France (11) and Portugal (6). The different rates indicate differences in definitions, legal systems and procedures. The study found that total numbers of compulsory admissions were increasing in Germany, France, England, Austria, Sweden and Finland, but this appeared to be balanced by an emphasis on shorter lengths of inpatient stay at the expense of more frequent re-admissions. The law of all EU member states stipulates that a confirmed mental disorder is a major condition for detention. However, it was found that additional criteria vary widely. Threatened or actual danger to oneself or others was the most common additional criterion, but this did not apply in Italy, Spain or Sweden. With regard to those countries which included the need for treatment in their procedures, Denmark, Finland, Greece, Ireland, Portugal and the UK regarded actual danger to oneself or others to be a sufficient criterion to warrant treatment on its own. Ten member states stipulated that the final decision on involuntary placement needed to be made by a non-medical authority. The remainder left the decision to psychiatrists or other health care professionals. It is significant that those states with the obligatory inclusion of a legal representative showed significantly lower compulsory admission rates. With regard to diagnostic patterns, again although the data is limited, 'schizophrenia' and related disorders were the predominant diagnosis in five out of nine of the countries surveyed where data was available. A tendency to compulsorily detain male patients more frequently than female patients was also noted in relation to Belgium, France, Ireland, Luxembourg and the Netherlands.

It is also useful to review parallel developments such as those taking place in Australia over the past fourteen years. As Fossey et al (2001) point out, the approach to setting the national health goals and targets which determine funding priorities and set in place outcome evaluation, had its origin in reforms to the NHS in the UK enacted by the Conservative government in the 1990s. The First National Mental Health Plan (1993–8) in Australia heralded a move away from long-stay mental health institutions towards locating psychiatric units within general hospitals. Emphasis was also placed on the co-ordination of hospital and community components of mental health services to provide a 'seamless' continuity of care.

The Second National Mental Health Plan (1998–2003) focused on mental health promotion, prevention – with attention being paid to depression as well as psychosis – the development of partnerships between agencies, and between the agencies and service users, the meeting of national standards, adherence to evidence-based practice, the development of measures of effectiveness and mental health workforce education and training initiatives. The National Standards for Mental Health Services have been presented in Australia as reflecting a strong commitment to values related to human rights, dignity and empowerment. They focus specifically on the accreditation of services, on supplying mechanisms for service monitoring and quality improvement, on providing a blueprint for service development, on informing consumers and carers about what to expect of a mental health service and on creating consumer and carer feedback mechanisms. In relation to Aboriginal people and Torres Strait Islanders there has been a particular emphasis on 'culturally appropriate outreach services' (Meadows and Singh 2002).

Although the implementation of these measures has varied from state to state, the similarities with the English system are clear. Accordingly the tension, paradox and inconsistency present in mental health policy and practice in England and Wales can be seen to have a wider-ranging relevance.

TENSION, PARADOX AND INCONSISTENCY

The picture presented is that New Labour has energetically tackled entrenched problems in the field of mental health. It has set in motion a comprehensive system of clinical governance which incorporates a systematic setting of standards with milestones and performance indicators and monitoring processes. It has emphasized the importance of training and professional self-regulation. It is trying to address recognized shortfalls in provision and resources. It has emphasized the value of 'joined-up' thinking and partnership working. It has taken steps to involve service users, paying particular attention to women and those from black and minority ethnic communities, and it has introduced measures to safeguard the public and to foster the social inclusion of those with mental health problems by means of welfare-to-work policies and the Disability Discrimination Act 1995. Is it surprising therefore that this ambitious programme contains inbuilt tension, paradox and inconsistency? It is also the case that new directives and initiatives have to be implemented in the context of prevailing policies, practices and organizational cultures. Within organizations or at grass-roots levels, those policies and practices which are seen to be working well or which fit particular organizational or service user cultures tend to be resistant to change. The new, or perhaps that which is being presented as new, is molded around the old like an extra layer of enamel on a worn tooth. In line with this analogy, the old will quickly cut through the new at points of greatest use. For both these reasons, tension, paradox and inconsistency are inevitable. Sometimes these result in insurmountable problems and the translation of a new policy initiative into practice fails or changes to become something completely different. At other times, tension, paradox and inconsistency can be put to good use and can produce policy-to-practice translations that are dynamic and which fit, in a similar way or in many different ways, with the interests of a wide variety of stakeholders. An examination of areas of tension, paradox and inconsistency includes the following: the opposing themes of managing risk and promoting social inclusion associated with the 'rights' and 'responsibilities' agenda of the government; the pull between local and centralized models of service delivery; evidence-based practice versus the tailoring of services to meet individual needs; and, to continue a theme introduced in Chapter 2, the various challenges posed to the prevailing medicalized mental health framework from those who have experience of mental distress. Throughout this chapter prevailing tension, paradox and inconsistency is also used as a means of constructively critiquing current policy.

The government's Social Exclusion Unit relatively belatedly turned its attention towards people with mental health difficulties. A consultation document (Office of the Deputy Prime Minister 2003) refers to the associated problems experienced by many people including long-term employment, poor physical health, alcohol and substance misuse and lasting social isolation. It also acknowledged the subsequent vicious circle which results from the mental health consequences of social exclusion. However, this emphasis can be seen to be at odds with the 'welfare-to-work' approach promoted by the government which emphasizes the value of work and the need to ensure access to training and employment. The tension between these policies can best be illustrated by looking at the way in which 'rights' have been associated with 'responsibilities'. In relation to this area the Labour government has clearly linked rights to responsibilities or obligations as part of its 'safe, sound and supportive' modernizing agenda (DOH 1998). By the enforced linking of responsibilities to rights, those unable to demonstrate responsibility by taking paid work can be denied rights and remain excluded. The state, by virtue of prevailing policies and legislation, has a duty of 'care' to this excluded group, but as always 'care' carries with it an element of control interpreted as safeguarding the vulnerable and protecting society from those assessed as dangerous or potentially dangerous. An emphasis on 'care' and 'control', which can include compulsion with regard to treatment, can be seen to sit uneasily with a concomitant stress on service user involvement and social inclusion (Fawcett, Featherstone and Goddard 2004). The reform of the Mental Health Act (1983), particularly those aspects relating to compulsory treatment in the community and the concomitant removal of the independent approved social worker role in the assessment process, renders involvement conditional upon the acceptance of non-negotiable pre-requisites. It is not impossible therefore to envisage a situation where access to those rights which are necessary to foster social inclusion is held conditional upon compliance with particular interventions and forms of treatment.

The concept of 'recovery' can also be linked to issues of social inclusion and has been the subject of government guidance. The document *Journey to Recovery* (DOH 2001b) states that mental health is one of the top three priorities for the government by means of the approach already set out in the *National Service Framework for Mental Health* (DOH 1999a) and *Modernising Mental Health Services* (DOH 1998). The emphasis on recovery is seen as an important aspect of challenging poor expectations and a negative outlook for people with difficulties and offers in their place a positive approach and a range of services to promote this, including an emphasis on employment and training issues and building self-respect and social networks within a framework of citizenship. However, there is again a tension with other strands of mental health policy which continue to place issues of risk and dangerousness centre stage with concomitant emphasis on conventional diagnosis/treatment patterns. There is also a lack of recognition that the concept of recovery itself is one which owes its origins to the service user movement. From this perspective there may be a challenge to the traditional bio-medical model and the need to move away from options of 'cure' or treatment in the conventional sense. According to Double (2002a), recovery is not about becoming 'symptom free', rather it is about reclaiming a socially valued life-style and the individual's control of the decisions she or he takes.

A related tension can be seen to lie at the heart of the current policy framework. The *National Service Framework for Mental Health* (DOH 1999a) as highlighted, focuses on seven key target areas. Progress in relation to these areas is measured by means of statistical returns, milestone and performance indicators. These forms of measurement sit uneasily with an associated emphasis on community involvement and patient forums. This is particularly the case if these strive to operate in a localized and democratic manner. As Goldie reports, 'the pressure to demonstrate achievement of National Service

Framework and other NHS targets often appears to be running counter to requirements for a locally developed service' (2003: 37). Goldie also emphasizes a priority slip in terms of the government's commitment to improving mental health services. Specifically he points to a narrow 'cost accountancy' perspective being applied to review the viability of schemes that require the acknowledgement of social costs and benefits, and highlights the ways in which the *National Service Framework* focuses on treatment rather than user-friendly and innovative forms of service development. This priority slip can also result in further tensions with regard to the allocation of resources, with money originally intended for mental health being spent on developing children's trusts or avoiding bed-blocking penalties.

Tensions are similarly apparent in relation to the emphasis placed on an inclusive integrated seamless service and the concomitant stress on a distinct national service framework with linked specific 'mental health' competencies to address each *National Service Framework* standard. There is something of a paradox between a strategy designed to promote inclusiveness and integration and an insistence on specialist mental health services working to specific criteria. Similarly, targeting services on particular groupings of service users can both resource an area and provide key services and at the same time exclude those who see themselves as experiencing 'mental ill-health' but who do not fit the specific service criteria.

There are corresponding inconsistencies in relation to the ways in which the government has promoted user and carer involvement in its policy documents. At one level user and carer involvement and participation may be demonstrated as a version of consumerism in terms of choice of services where the usual options of voice and exit may be all that is available (Hirschman in Hugman 1998). At the other end of the spectrum, user-led services may offer a vision of a model for the future where the planning and delivery are entirely within the remit of a service user group or organization. Models of service user and carer involvement may be placed along a continuum between these two extremes and may variously refer to the involvement of any individual in determining her or his own care or treatment plan or the representation of service users and carers by service users and carers within the planning, commissioning or management of services. Much has been written concerning the rhetoric and practice of the latter arrangements and how far service users and carers can participate on an equal basis and the ways in which their input can be marginalized or tokenized with scant recognition in terms of payment or access to support. This area is explored in greater detail in Chapter 6. However, it is important to note at this point that the apparent incorporation of user perspectives within service planning and service delivery forums can serve to remove the critical edge from user and carer groups at a time when rights are being subsumed into demonstrations of responsibility and the safety of those without mental health difficulties is being prioritized.

With regard to professional roles and identities within the field of mental health, it is obvious that in line with 'modernizing' imperatives, roles and tasks are changing, combining and evolving. Recommendations from *Pulling Together* (Sainsbury Centre for Mental Health [SCMH] 1997b) and the subsequent report *The Capable Practitioner* (SCMH 2000), include the retention of existing specialisms and professional roles, but strongly emphasize the need for greater levels of multi-disciplinary and shared training. Currently, close attention is being paid to the roles and responsibilities of the various professional groups within the workforce and the need to identify both the core competencies which underpin the work of all the disciplines involved as well as the specific and distinctive contribution required of each profession.

These changes again bring to the fore a variety of competing priorities and concerns. Many workers, for example, fear becoming de-skilled and sidelined as a result of these reforms. In relation to social workers, for example, there are limited opportunities to undertake further training apart from that associated with becoming an approved social worker and this is now changing. Community mental health nurses are also concerned that their hard-fought-for role combining clinical practice with a diverse range of social skills, will become narrower. The current agenda for the future of mental health professionals contains a number of diverse and uncertain scenarios. One of these relates to increasing the regulation and standardization of practice following the introduction of National Occupational Standards. The increasing regulation of the workforce is an area explored in greater depth in Chapter 7. However, while a focus on National Occupational Standards, national curricula and increased target setting, performance management and inspections, can maintain national standards and ensure uniformity, these measures can also be interpreted as moulding mental health professionals into technicians, where they can easily become mere rote followers of procedures, rather than reflective practitioners capable of working in partnership with others and utilizing vision and initiative.

As part of its modernizing strategy, the government has demonstrated a commitment to evidence-based practice, and has prioritized particular forms of interventions. There is a strong adherence to medicalized understandings of mental health, but also a move to make intervention strategies more broadly based. In relation to services for people diagnosed as suffering from psychoses, for example, psychosocial interventions and cognitive behavioural techniques have been promoted. As with many of New Labour's policy initiatives, the promotion of particular intervention strategies can be seen to be double-edged. On the one hand the use of different forms of intervention for a grouping previously regarded as resistant to any form of treatment apart from drug therapy is clearly a positive move. However, on the other, these forms of interventions focus on clear-cut managed solutions to problems that are in turn simplified and categorized. Wilson and Beresford (2002) highlight the difficulties that can result for the individual of making mental distress fit categories and classifications. The simplifying and standardizing of some of these therapeutic approaches for wider use, also opens up the possibility of increasing rigidity in application and of particular techniques becoming the new orthodoxy. This has taken place in relation to the promotion within the Probation Service of specific cognitive techniques, where procedures relating to the method to be used take precedence over attention to the process and the tailoring of the method to the needs of particular individuals in specific contexts.

It has also become apparent that, despite claims for evidence to inform practice, research evidence is ignored when it runs counter to political directives. As has been noted, public anxiety has been fuelled by a series of events highlighted in the media concerning the consequences of de-institutionalization and the shortcomings of 'community care' services. The deaths of Zito, Newby and Schwartz among others, and the media coverage of such events, have contributed to a climate of fear and unease towards those people with mental health difficulties living in the community. However, as we have seen in Chapter 3, research findings have shown that proportionally very small numbers of homicides, particularly homicides carried out on strangers, are committed by people diagnosed as having mental illness (Boyd 1994; Taylor and Gunn 1999). It would appear to be a media-driven association of mental illness with dangerousness which has informed the thinking behind many of the reforms proposed, rather than research evidence. This in turn calls into question the modernizing agenda's preoccupation with standards, targets, clinical governance and above all evidence-based practice reinforced by the National Institute for Clinical Excellence, the Institute for Evidence Based Practice and the parallel development of the Social Care Institute for Excellence. A key question to pose is whether the basis for reform is 'evidence' or event-driven media and public opinion. This can be allied to the thorny question of who determines what constitutes 'evidence' and who decides which 'evidence' is to be used to inform policy and practice. The National Institute for Mental Health in England (NIMHE 2003b) emphasizes allegiance to a hierarchy of evidence as utilized in the *National Service Framework of Mental Health* (DOH 1999a) which privileges systematic reviews and randomized controlled trials, and subsumes the qualitative beneath the quantitative with associated implication for quality. Cooper (2003) also concludes in his appraisal of evidence-based policy in mental health, that despite evidence-based health care being promulgated as a rational basis for mental health planning in Britain, only 10% of the clinical trials and meta-analyses which he surveyed actually focused on the effectiveness of services and many of the studies proved inconclusive. Furthermore, the notion of evidence-based practice has been seen as fundamentally antithetical to partnership working with service users. Frost suggests that: 'If we do indeed base all our practice on "evidence", then by default any room for negotiation, partnership and compromise with the service user is lost' (2002: 50).

Additional tensions can be identified in the current emphasis on public/private finance initiatives. Public/private financing schemes are justified on the basis that they reflect the new mixed economy promoted by 'third way' politics. These initiatives and associated policies, it is argued, will create a synergy between public and private sectors by utilizing the perceived dynamism of the markets whilst at the same time keeping the public interest in mind (Giddens 1998). However, again, the tension created by the need to prioritize public accountability in public/private endeavours and the overall complexity imbedded in the public sector which makes it difficult to apply direct single-issue private sector solutions to multi-issue public sector problems, are embedded in the policy. Evidence that public/ private finance initiatives have not lived up to their promotional billing in the public sector (e.g. Monbiot 2001), despite, as emphasized, the much-publicized concern with evidence and evidence-based practice in relation to social work, social care and health, also appears to have been ignored. In relation to mental health, public/private finance initiatives raise two key questions. The first relates to the attractiveness of this area for private finance and the second clearly focuses on the ways in which business pressures can take precedence over the interests of service users.

CONCLUDING REMARKS

The government by means of the 'modernizing' agenda aims to make mental health services 'safe, sound and supportive' (DOH 1998). Emphasis is placed on social inclusion, prevention and 'joined-up thinking' allied to a specific focus on joint planning, commissioning, service delivery and the meeting of specific targets. However, in line with the perspectives and debates discussed in Chapters 2 and 3, the White Paper *Modernising Mental Health Services* (1998), the *National Service Framework for Mental Health* (DOH 1999a), the reform of the 1983 Mental Health Act, and the Health and Social Care Act (2001), there can be seen to be a reaffirmation of the dominance of medicalized and clinical constructions of 'mental health' within social policy and practice in England and Wales. This view is re-inforced by the emphasis placed in these legislative and policy documents on the management of mental illness by assessing risk and providing treatment and care more quickly and conveniently, rather than upon ways of breaking down oppressive barriers and enabling excluded and categorized groupings of people to become fully participating citizens.

The areas discussed emphasize the tension, paradox and inconsistency apparent in the application of current government policy. The highlighting of these areas serves both as a means of facilitating constructive critique and as a way of drawing attention to productive aspects. The juxtaposing of different agendas can create space to manoeuvre and to bring about challenge and change. It can also prevent particular policies being rigidly applied in practice to the detriment of innovation and regional prioritizations.

The changing contemporary scene: forwards–backwards

6 User/survivor involvement and 'carers'

> We are all the primary experts on our own mental health, and about what works for us. We are more than the sum of our individual problems and of the services that we use. We can and should value and appreciate the coping strategies we have developed for ourselves.
>
> (The Mental Health Foundation [TMHF] 1997: 7)

This chapter takes forward some of the issues raised in previous chapters, explores the history and the development of the survivor movement and considers the impact of this movement in the field of mental health. The early fragmented nature of the survivor movement in the UK, the influence of developments elsewhere and the links with the Disability Rights Movement are examined and the commonalities as well as the differences are noted. In particular, the development and application of the social model of disability, initially developed in respect of physical disability and subsequently related to mental illness, is explored. The increasing recruitment of people with experience of service use to work in mental health services is additionally reviewed and the varied perspectives on involvement, which may include campaigning, the development of user-led services, as well involvement in current service developments, are appraised. Finally, the notion of 'citizenship' is subject to critical interrogation.

CONSUMERISM, CONSULTATION AND 'EMPOWERMENT': THE OLD ARGUMENTS

Consumer choice as a key policy platform surged into the limelight with the 1989 White Paper *Caring for People: Community Care in the Next Decade and Beyond* (DOH 1989) which informed the NHS and Community Care Act (1990). The changes outlined at this time were intended to 'give people a greater individual say in how they live their lives and the services they need to help them to do so'. 'Promoting choice and independence' became a major slogan of the Conservative government of the time (1989: para 1.8.5).

Although consumer choice initially sounded like a 'good thing' and a positive move, contemporary analysts questioned whether needs and services could be commodified and made accessible to individuals in the manner described. Fiona Williams (1992) drew attention to the fact that the control of resources by social services departments clearly diminished the negotiating power of individuals both in terms of choice and with regard to how community care packages operated. Similarly the promotion of an 'active consumer' approach failed to take account of the mediation of a third agency and the inability of most 'consumers' to meet their own needs out of their own resources.

Dissatisfaction with notions of consumerism led to the term 'empowerment' being used as the panacea to address power differentials between service users and professionals and to highlight issues of rights and entitlements. However, the term became devalued by the way it was employed to describe and also to justify a whole variety of different approaches, processes and end products. Oliver (1996) from the perspective of the Disability Rights Movement criticized those who regarded 'empowerment' as a thing or an entity. He emphasized that empowerment could only be viewed as a process and one that necessitated clarity and ongoing negotiation. Croft and Beresford (1992) and Beresford and Croft (1993) tried to revalue 'empowerment' by defining 'consultation' and 'empowerment' more clearly and precisely and by detailing the steps which needed to be taken by all participants to formulate empowering strategies and processes. They defined 'consultation' as an agency-led, top-down attempt to elicit service users and carers comments and recommendations, and 'empowerment' as service user and/or carer-led initiatives to obtain autonomy and power. Necessary features included agency commitment at principle and policy level, an agreement to continually review 'working together' practices and procedures, joint training opportunities, the availability of appropriate resources, ongoing clarity about what is on offer, the ongoing negotiation of outcomes and the facilitation of an environment which presents positive images of people and encourages reciprocity and exchange. Fawcett and Featherstone (1996) in turn queried whether 'empowerment', as defined in Croft and Beresford (1992) and Beresford and Croft (1993) was a process which professionals, agencies and service users could jointly and actively facilitate. They suggested that the conflicts, the tensions and the possibility of appropriation (Dowson 1990; Baistow 1995) were such that empowering processes were unlikely to be effective if responsibility continued to rest primarily with professionals and agencies. They indicated that 'empowering' initiatives needed to be reinforced by service user groups operating outside agency structures actively negotiating and campaigning on behalf of their own agendas. However, despite problems with definition and debates about who should be involved in the process, 'empowerment' has continued to be used to describe various kinds of participative activity ranging from basic consultation, to active listening (which may then result in action, inaction or appropriation), to a collective, user-led struggle against discrimination and oppression.

TERMINOLOGY

As discussed in the Introduction, terminology is important and labels easily become entrenched and associated with particular meanings, divisions and power relationships. With regard to those who use services, currently 'service user' or 'user' is the most commonly used term, although 'survivor' is gaining momentum. Older terms such as 'client' or 'patient' continue to be widely used and many people in receipt of services have no choice but to respond to the label that custom and practice, in particular settings, have caused to become commonplace. However, when individuals choose a label, as Wallcraft and Bryant (2003) acknowledge, the term used often reflects personal experiences. They point out that those choosing to use 'survivor' tend, for example, to be more challenging of medicalized understandings of mental health, whilst those employing the term 'user' tend to see working with or within the system as the way forward. This apparent distinction can be illustrated by the debate in *OpenMind* in March/April 2003 between the case for retaining day centres 'that work for us' (Excell and Mayes 2003: 26) and the argument that such provision is outmoded and unhelpful and should be abolished (Perkins 2003). Excell and Mayes (2003) maintain: 'Now that we have places to meet that work for us, why advocate getting rid of them? Far better to work towards changing the aspects that don't work and tailoring the services to meet all of our needs' (Excell and Mayes 2003: 26). Others have exercised choice to devise their own name. Michael Elvin, for example, writes in *Community Care* magazine of the decision of those using a social services day centre to call themselves 'consumerees'. He states:

> By deciding a name for ourselves we liberate ourselves. Consumerees dismiss claims that we are being empowered – instead we resist attempts to disempower us from the start. And consumerees are not afraid of jargon, but ask and challenge when appropriate.
>
> (Elvin 2003: 22)

Undoubtedly, setting choice against imposed orthodoxies serves to polarize the discussion and also raises the issue about whether group labels are ever appropriate given the ease with which certain labels can be devalued and those holding these labels categorized and classified. Within disability and mental health movements, as highlighted in Chapter 2, many have chosen to revalue previously devalued labels such as 'mad' and 'cripple' and to positively challenge negative categorizations, asserting the importance of difference and diversity. There is also the matter of positive imagery to consider. The stigma attached to mental health problems is such that those who have positive images to offer are often reluctant to come forward. Perkins (2003) maintains that it is essential to keep 'hope and opportunity' alive. She states:

> Mental health opportunity must be about this goal: helping people to live the lives they want to lead. And in the service of this, hope and opportunity are central. The professionals' core role must be to help people to hold on to hope and access the opportunities they seek . . . and we still have a long way to go.
>
> (Perkins 2003: 6)

In this chapter the term 'user/survivor' will be used to reflect the range of positions currently occupied, from 'challenge and change' to retaining 'what works for us'. In other chapters, the terms used reflect the topic being discussed. As part of this discussion, it is also useful to highlight that we all move in and out of different groups with different labels; some of these can be seen to be pejorative, some neutral, some status-enhancing. We are also continually, both actively and passively, rejecting and accepting such labels. This is not to negate the previous discussion, but to acknowledge that this is a universal issue and not one that solely relates to an identified minority.

USER/SURVIVOR MOVEMENTS

As discussed in Chapter 3, the history of challenge and resistance to the more coercive and controlling aspects of mental health care is one that is frequently overlooked. Peter Campbell (1996) refers to a long-established tradition of a user/survivor movement. He highlights that there has always been a protest from people at their treatment by society including 'The Petition of the Poor Distracted People in the House of Bedlam' (1620) and attempts in the nineteenth century to counter the negative care in the asylums, such as the Alleged Lunatics' Friends Society formed in 1845 by John Perceval and others, with Perceval having written of his own experiences in the asylums. This was continued by those who spoke out about their experiences of being treated for shell shock after the First World War or who were given electroconvulsive therapy (ECT) in the 1930s and 1940s. The Mental Patients Union was created in the early 1970s and the anti-psychiatry movement also led to groups forming such as the British Network for Alternatives to Psychiatry. In 1985 an international conference, held in Brighton, drew attention to the fragmented nature of user activity in the UK and that same year the MIND conference for the first time included substantial input from survivors in workshops and plenary sessions. As the pace of change accelerated, by the mid-1990s there were over 350 local, regional and national groups.

With regard to challenging entrenched conceptualizations and pressing for change, the disability movement has a thirty-year history of 'against the odds' achievement. It has achieved a sea change in the way that disability is understood since Paul Hunt took a stance at Le Court Cheshire Home against the entrenched position of the management group and the findings of researchers Miller and Gwynne in 1972 (see Finkelstein 1991: 19–39). The view that people are disabled by oppressive social, political, economic and cultural constructs, rather than by individual impairments, and the campaign for full citizenship rights and social inclusion, are now firmly entrenched in mainstream thinking. The Disability Discrimination Act (DDA) (1995) and the Disability Rights Commission, although continuing to have shortcomings, a medicalized orientation and exclusionary clauses, have made it illegal to discriminate against disabled people. Legislation following the Draft Disability Bill (2004) further challenges discrimination in relation to access and transport. Those with mental health problems are included in the disability statistics and are to some extent covered by the legislation,[1] but the relationship between the user/survivor movement and the disability movement has tended to be an uneasy one.

The user/survivor movement is seen as having a more recent origin than the disability movement although, as has already been noted, there are numerous historical examples of resistance to coercive and oppressive care. Both movements contain adherents who are reluctant to claim allegiance to the other. Reasons include the need to reclaim different identities and to prioritize different areas, such as the right to physical access as opposed to the abolition of compulsory treatment. The ways in which personal experiences differ, with the needs of users/survivors perhaps being more episodic, have also created barriers. However, the similarities associated with the need for individual control, the importance of challenging discrimination and oppression, the need to tackle specific disabling measures, such as those associated with the benefits system, and the ongoing campaign for rights and full citizenship, have persuaded many users/survivors to make links with the disability movement in order to enhance the impact and bargaining power of both movements.

The user/survivor movement in the UK gained momentum in the early 1980s when local user forums were established on a nationwide basis. This movement was stimulated by contact with Dutch and US groups and by the promotion of user-led advocacy. Wallcraft and Bryant in 2003 surveyed the extent and scope of the mental health user/survivor movement in the

---

1 The extent to which those with mental health problems are covered by DDA (1995) and the criteria used in the DDA (1995) to determine if someone is disabled are related to the individual's ability to carry out day-to-day activities and these are defined in terms of physical capacities such as the ability to walk, etc. In relation to mental health (unlike physical impairments) there also has to be a clinical diagnosis and the problem has to be seen as long-term and enduring.

UK.[2] They also endeavoured to ascertain the degree to which existing groups represented the wider constituency of service users and survivors, including those from minority ethnic groups. Overall, the survey identified 300 groups which were seen to have common beliefs and understandings and which overall could be seen to form a movement. It was found that these groups were involved in a wide range of activities moving from statutory consultation in local service planning and development, to offering mutual support, to combating stigma and facilitating 'recovery', to helping people experiencing mental distress avoid using statutory services. White men were seen to be well represented although women, and black women in particular, did not report positive experiences of their issues being taken up by local groups. Black people generally were not seen to be particularly well represented, although it was found that some national networks were making clear efforts to involve black and minority ethnic service users. However, the survey found that most groups tended to have a small membership, to be recently formed and to have insecure and limited funding. There was also seen to be a lack, at national level, of a national forum to bring together the various service user networks.

As noted earlier, within the broad range of groups in the user movement, there is, to some extent, a distinction to be made between those who are concerned with working to effect change within existing mainstream services, and those who align themselves more closely with a radical rather than reformist agenda, seeking to provide alternative sources of support which are user-managed, -led and -delivered (Perkins and Repper 1998).

The growth of user/survivor groups has also promoted the development of user involvement in research and also user-led research projects. The Nuffield Foundation (1997), for example, has provided guidance on involving users. This emphasizes the importance of not treating users as objects of investigation, of ensuring that the research project has an agreed and clear value base and of articulating a clear involvement strategy that takes account of resource issues, training needs and reimbursement. Moore, Beazley and Maelzer (1998) advocate a reflexive, self-analytical and critical approach to disability research firmly grounded in human

2 Significant user networks in the UK include the UK Advocacy Network (UKAN), which is a national network for service user-led advocacy projects and local user forums; Survivors Speak Out (SSO), a group formed initially for service users and professional allies; the National Voices Network (NVN), which operates within Rethink, formerly the National Schizophrenia Fellowship; the Hearing Voices Network, which has 150 groups and focuses on positive ways of coping with hearing voices. Other groups include Mindlink, which is a consultative body to ensure that users/survivors have a direct say in shaping MIND's policy campaigns; No Panic, which is a user-led voluntary organization that aims to help those experiencing anxiety-related problems; Mad Pride, which is a political campaigning group wanting to positively reclaim and re-evaluate mental health.

rights principles. They stress the need to go beyond 'partnership approaches' and state:

> . . . the notion of partnership may constitute the latest bandwagon for well-meaning, enthusiastic groups of disabled people and their non-disabled allies seeking to research together. We are in favour of a partnership approach that brings disabled and non-disabled people together, but are trying to place it within a stronger framework which has critical reflection on human rights as its foundation . . . all will not simply be well just because disabled people and non-disabled people conduct research together; integrity and credibility have to be carefully established in relation to both academic rigour and political commitments.
>
> (Moore, Beazley and Maelzer 1998: 94)

In terms of user/survivor-led research, the Users' Voices Project (Rose 2001) provides an interesting example and was promoted and funded by the Sainsbury Centre for Mental Health (SCMH). It is significant because it outlines how a user-led approach can be developed in such a way that it can be rolled out to different areas and because the findings powerfully reinforce the views emanating from other user/survivor groups. The model used is called user-focused monitoring and it involves a project co-ordinator, who is also usually a service user/survivor with research skills, recruiting group members from local day centres, work projects and survivor groups. This group then works on producing a questionnaire, a site visitors workbook or a set of focus group questions and formulating a set of 'core' questions, which are then reviewed and amended by subsequent groups. Group members are trained in interviewing techniques and focus group co-ordination. A pilot study is carried out before the interviewers move on to the main data collection exercise and, to ensure that individuals who are very isolated are included, the sample population is identified on a random basis. Feedback from the interviews is discussed at group meetings and the project co-ordinator analyses the data with the groups, promoting discussion of the findings.

The techniques described above are not particularly innovative, but in a similar way to approaches reviewed by the Nuffield Institute (2001) work effectively and do have, in terms of questions posed, data collected, findings produced and dissemination activities, an emphasis that significantly differs from research which is professionally directed. There are always questions to be asked about the role of the experienced project co-ordinator *vis-à-vis* the service users groups, but this is clearly a way of operating which takes research process issues fully into account.

However, user/survivor involvement in research is not without its risks. These can be seen as relating to the marginalization of such research within the wider arena where evidence-based practice holds sway and the possible appropriation of knowledge by professionals. In terms of the former, Faulkner and Thomas (2002) point to the 'dominance of neuroscience' and a level of 'political resistance to seeing psychiatric patients as experts and . . . partners in setting research agendas' (2002: 1). Within this, traditional research in terms of the gold standard inherent in randomized controlled trials, conventional funding and an emphasis on symptomology, has, as yet, to be seriously challenged by user-led research which highlights subjective experiences and the quality of people's everyday lives. Equally, the voices and experiences of service users, heralded in policy documents such as *Modernising Mental Health Services* (DOH 1998) and *The NHS Plan* (DOH 2000b) as being of importance, remain relegated to the margins of research in comparison with other forms of 'evidence'. As pointed out by Beresford (2003b), this means that those who have the experience are seen as unreliable and too subjective in their knowledge and can always be regarded as being in the weakest position to tell it reliably. Instead he argues that the opposite may be true and that 'the greater the distance between knowledge or evidence and the direct experience on which it is based, then the more likely that knowledge or evidence is to be unreliable, inaccurate or distorted'. The solution proposed by Faulkner and Thomas requires 'A marriage of two types of expertise . . . expertise by experience and expertise by profession' (2002: 3).

With regard to the appropriation of user/survivor knowledge and experience by academics, professionals and researchers, this can be seen as an ongoing site of contestation. Drawing on the concept of 'cultural capital' outlined by Bourdieu as the dominant culture and the currency through which power can be attained and conventionally applied to explain class differences in educational achievement, the lived experience of users/survivors has come to be seen as valuable currency in itself. With regard to social work theory, Beresford (2000) has referred to the traditional model whereby user/survivor knowledge is interpreted and mediated by academics and professionals and suggests that this cannot continue unquestioned. Instead, users/survivors must be centrally involved and included in the process of developing theory and knowledge and mediating experience. This approach directly challenges conventional notions of neutrality in line with feminist critiques of traditional research and inquiry which reject the notion of universal truth and instead focus on the reflexive interrogation of different positionings from which there may be many different 'truths'. The continuing location of users/survivors as only 'subjects' of research rather than as active participants, or the exploitation of networks and contacts, can no longer be justified. Whilst the cruder examples of exploitative and oppressive research strategies may no longer occur, there is a continuing risk that experiences similar to those identified by feminist researchers, whereby user/survivor researchers are seen as inferior and historical imbalances of power continue, are maintained (Rose 2003).

THE PROCESS OF CHANGE

There are indications that change is occurring in relation to user/survivor involvement in mental health services, although on a smaller scale and at a slower pace than envisaged. As we have seen, current policy documents, such as *Modernising Mental Health Services* (DOH 1998), emphasize the need for patients, service users and carers to be involved in their own care and in planning services. The increasing voice of service users and carers is being articulated through a variety of formal and informal mechanisms. Community involvement is now on the agenda in NHS trusts, primary care trusts, health and social care trusts, social services departments and voluntary and private organizations. To be effective, user involvement requires attention at a number of levels including that of involvement in individual care plans and delivery, involvement in team and service issues, strategic involvement in the design and development of services as well as involvement in research and evaluation. The range of consultative and participatory initiatives available, as highlighted, clearly varies between the different organizations and services, but the fact that there is now a clear remit to ensure that the views of service users and carers are sought with regard to new developments and existing services as well as in relation to training and education initiatives, has to be regarded as constructive.

Additionally, service users are becoming involved in contributing to the direct provision of services. Service users, employed as patients' advocates, and support workers are found within community mental health teams and there are also examples of user-led initiatives in relation to crisis services and informal support groups.

The development and application of the notion of 'recovery' as a concept conceived of by survivors rather than by professionals as indicated in Chapter 5 also represent a significant and influential move forward in the field of mental health. A recovery-oriented approach is one which is able to

> support an individual in their own personal development, building self-esteem, identity and finding a meaningful role in society.
>
> (Allott and Loganathan 2002: 4)

However, whilst concepts such as 'recovery' and the application of the social model of disability, drawn from the physical disability movement, to mental health, owe their origins to the work of service users and survivors, these are increasingly being claimed within mainstream policy and are at risk of losing their radical potential for change. Instead a sanitized version is promulgated which may bear little relation to the power of the original. For example, the recent government document entitled *Journey to Recovery* (DOH 2001b), although maintaining a positive approach, provides an overview of existing policy with little reference to the concept of recovery as defined by individual service users.

There is also an increasing level of involvement of service users/survivors and carers in the training and education of mental health workers, although again progress is uneven and variable ranging from non-involvement, limited involvement in terms of consultation and limited curricular input, to a higher level of collaboration or partnership where involvement is embedded throughout the process of curriculum design, delivery, assessment and review. User and carer involvement has been increasingly promoted by professional bodies and funders, with, for example, the General Social Care Council (GSCC), the regulatory body for social work in England, stipulating that stakeholder involvement is an essential element in the design and development of the new social work qualification. The guidance states that programmes must ensure that stakeholder representatives, particularly service users and employers, are involved in the selection of students (DOH 2002b) and the criteria for accreditation require the involvement of service users and other stakeholders in the design, delivery and monitoring of courses (GSCC 2002). More broadly across mental health education, quality improvement tools are being introduced, such as one produced by the Northern Centre for Mental Health (Brooker, James and Redhead 2003) based on Goss and Miller's framework (1995), and designed to contribute to the development of systematic and strategic approaches to user and carer involvement in education and training. The employment of lecturing staff with experience of mental health difficulties, as opposed to visiting speakers, which has occurred in some institutions, will also have an impact.

However, despite these positive shifts, which include the appointment of a disability rights activist as the Social Care Institute for Excellence's chairperson in 2002, the overall picture relating to general service user involvement remains mixed. In terms of findings, the Users' Voice Project (Rose 2001), referred to earlier, found that mental health service users require more information on a range of issues in order for them to be *involved in* rather than *recipients of* mental health care. Users/survivors reported that the Care Programme Approach (CPA) did not appear to be working in that the majority of users did not know what the CPA was, who their key workers were or whether they had a care plan. Additionally, most users/survivors felt that their 'needs' were identified by professionals as problems and that their strengths and abilities were not considered. When asked what was missing from their care many said they wanted someone to talk to about ordinary things and someone to lend a sympathetic ear. Perceptions of discharge were not positive and many did not know whom to contact if they experienced a mental health crisis. With regard to medication, whilst many clearly stated that they suffered from the side effects of psychotropic drugs, many also appreciated the effects of the drugs on the reduction of symptoms. However, it became clear that male black users were still more likely to receive medication by injection than white service users. The findings clearly showed that users did not feel involved in making decisions about their care at any level. The report states: 'It is clear that the government's intention of putting the patient "at the centre" has not filtered down to all those who provide mental health services – be they organizations or individual mental health professionals' (Users' Voices Project, Rose 2001: 7).

Similarly, the survey carried out by Wallcraft and Bryant (2003) demonstrates that, despite ways forward being clearly identified, little has changed on the ground. They point out that although their survey found 72% of local user/survivor-led mental health groups represented on local planning forums, this did not appear to be leading to significant changes in service provision. They found that low priority tended to be given to user-led projects and little flexibility accorded to the priorities of user representatives, such as advocacy projects or minority ethnic user groups. Similarly money did not appear to have been made available for the voluntary sector or for expanding and improving local services. It also needs to be borne in mind that the process of involvement itself can, if negative responses are received, cause distress. Harrison (2002) reports that many users/survivors were quizzed about their motives and asked to justify their representativeness. Many also reported a lack of clarity regarding payment, and many commented on sheer exhaustion from being repeatedly called upon by agencies who wanted to demonstrate compliance with user representation targets. In this respect, the potential for tokenism may also increase, as there is increasing emphasis on user involvement as a performance indicator for quality assurance or bench-marking purposes.

With regard to service users working in partnership with professionals, the tension between the power held by professionals and the ways in which this can be and has been challenged or ameliorated by those who have experience of mental distress, is a pertinent one. It is also clear that there are still many service users who do not have access to partnership initiatives, and agencies and professionals who are unfamiliar and sometimes uncomfortable with this changing perspective. The situation in relation to African-Caribbean communities as cited above also warrants specific attention.

Barnes and Bowl (2001) continue to highlight the complexity of notions such as 'partnership' and shared decision-making between professionals and service users/survivors. They draw attention to the way in which the power of professionals is maintained through its continued manifestation within the rules and processes of consultation and participation. The means by which professionals can intentionally or unintentionally subvert professional/user/survivor partnership arrangements or involvement in service management and service planning are well documented and have been referred to earlier (e.g. Baistow 1994; Fawcett and Featherstone 1996). Organizations such as the SCMH and The Mental Health Foundation (TMHF) have argued for specific measures to redress the balance. These include ensuring that professionals in purchasing and providing capacities facilitate rather than control user involvement, that resources are clearly linked to the provision of finance, that attention is paid to user training issues and that the fragile infrastructures of user/survivor groups are supported. The necessity of making sure that planning and management procedures are transparent and accessible is also reiterated. It is highlighted that the measurement of the extent of user involvement at all levels has to clearly relate to the extent to which users themselves feel involved, rather than to external measures. The importance of users/survivors being placed at the centre of the monitoring and evaluation of mental health services, with particular attention being paid to issues relating to gender, sexuality and ethnicity, is also emphasized (Rose 2001; TMHF 2001).

Finally, amongst the many aspects and issues related to the process of user/survivor involvement it is easy to lose sight of the desired outcomes and impact of involvement on services. A review of the impact of user involvement in social care, including mental health, learning disability, services for older people as well as children and young people, undertaken by the Social Care Institute for Excellence, indicates that:

> The true effectiveness of these processes to promote user-led change and impact on service improvement remains largely untested.
>
> (Carr 2004: 8)

The review refers to the relatively weak evidence base for the impact of user involvement on organizational change (Rose et al 2003). There is also the view that user involvement should be seen primarily as having a therapeutic purpose rather than contributing to a shift in the balance of power between users and professionals/organizations. Whilst it is important not to underestimate the personal value of involvement and the contribution to recovery in terms of increased self-esteem, confidence, access into voluntary work and employment, failure to acknowledge the need to address power imbalances can only be counterproductive. Meaningful involvement can be multifaceted. One participant in a study of women's experiences of mental health services in one city stated that her involvement in the project had

> handed back to me a feeling of being in control which, when taken away from us in our illness, contributes to keeping us in decline.
>
> (Resistors 2002: 23)

It is also important to re-emphasize that those groups who are marginalized from mainstream services can also face difficulties within a predominantly white heterosexual user movement.

Understandings of mental health and experiences of the current system affect whether users/survivors want to work with professionals or to campaign separately and on their own terms. The Disability Rights Movement has demonstrated the power and influence which can be wielded by disabled people coming together to promote a particular political, civil and rights-based programme supported by a radical, yet accessible, conceptualization of disability This has effectively changed the focus of attention from disabled individuals to a disabling society that actively disables people with impairments. The Disability Rights Movement has accepted non-disabled adherents of the social model of disability as part of its campaign to change legislation, policy and practice, but the spearhead of the movement has been, controversially at times, those with experience of disability. There will continue to be those who believe that the way forward lies in survivors campaigning outside of the current system. There will be those who want to engage with what is on offer and develop and improve it. There will also continue to be a whole variety of positions in between.

THE FAMILY AND CARERS

In moving on to consider the part played by carers and their involvement within the wider canvas of mental health, it quickly becomes apparent that there are a number of tensions and dilemmas. Not the least of these is the now-historical assumption, prevalent in the mid-twentieth century, that families are to blame as causal agents in the development of mental health problems. More recently a crude reversal of this belief can be found in the notion that carers are the selfless and self-sacrificing heroes and heroines who shoulder the 'burden' of care. What is clear, however, is evidence of the increasing recognition of the importance of the role played by carers and the need for appropriate support, rights and benefits, enshrined in legislation and policy guidance.

Any analysis of these issues therefore necessarily requires a closer examination of power relationships, a critical review of the discourse of 'caring' and the need to locate changing historical trends within the wider ideological and political environment. It is notable that in the 1970s, explanations of serious mental illness relied heavily on either biological explanations or models of faulty and damaging early family relationships. This contributed to the paradox that either families have little part to play in support and recovery or they are to blame for the ill-health of one of their members. The latter view was supported by the writings of Laing (1965) underpinned by sociological critiques of the family then prevalent. Now that this view is recognized as unhelpful and unproven, an alternative view seeks to position families and carers as partners in the provision of support and treatment and there is an emphasis on family involvement which includes education and training. One particular aspect of this approach is a concern that high levels of 'expressed emotion' within the family environment contribute to the maintenance of symptoms and intervention is aimed at helping family members to spend less time together and to develop practical ways of resolving problems and difficulties within the home (Leff and Vaughan 1981; Dixon and Lehman 1995). There is, however, a continuing debate as to the distinction between maintenance and causation of illness (Johnstone 2000). It is also perhaps relevant to note the increased importance of bringing a positive model of family and informal caring support into an environment where the emphasis is on community rather than institutional care, a move at least partially fuelled, as previously discussed, by the soaring costs of hospital and residential provision.

Closer working with families, however, may also raise other tensions whereby the affirmation of informal carers, alongside professionals as partners in the provision of care and support, may serve to re-enforce the powerlessness and one-dimensional role experienced by service users. Indeed the term 'carer' undermines the autonomy of those experiencing mental distress. Many writers from within the disability movement have drawn attention to how this term assumes a uni-dimensional relationship between those referred to as 'the carer' and 'the cared for' and ignores that caring relationships are multi-dimensional and reciprocal. Morris (1993) and Corker and French (1999) amongst others have challenged the invisibility of those given the label of 'cared for' and who are seen as 'other' and subordinate, both victim and incapable, a 'burden' on their care-givers (Shakespeare 2000). The prevailing emphasis on the needs of carers, for example, as specified within Standard 6 of the *National Service Framework for Mental Health* (DOH 1999a), whilst important at one level, not only mixes together the needs of 'users and carers' but also fails to acknowledge the complexity of social and emotional relationships and the potential tensions and differences in needs and perspectives. This point is emphasized by Sayce who comments that her relationship with a partner with a diagnosis of manic depression does not make her a 'carer' because:

> This is a mutual relationship, not one in which 'care' goes one way, and not one involving 'burden' (an offensive term that should be dropped from research design and discussion).
>
> (Sayce 2000: 11)

She continues that such a relationship can also lead to other forms of discrimination and stigma including personal concerns about the motivation for such relationships and that such matters are rarely publicly discussed. The role of people with mental health difficulties themselves as carers or involved in mutual and reciprocal relationships is itself rarely considered and can be seen as further evidence of the dichotomized thinking which permeates both policy and practice.

Notwithstanding such concerns, as well as the possible confusion between formal and informal relationships and some suggestion that the term 'personal assistant' may be regarded as more appropriate, 'carer' remains the common term used in everyday speech as well as in government documents and reports. It is used in this chapter, but the critiques are fully acknowledged and taken on board.

In addition to the tensions and pitfalls inherent in the involvement of carers and their recognition as partners alongside professionals *vis-à-vis* users/survivors, there is also a need to move beyond the rhetoric of 'caring for carers' as for many appropriate support continues to remain illusory and beyond reach. On the one hand they may experience a range of difficulties which can include social isolation, tiredness, the loss of friends and relationships and mental health difficulties in their own right (Hogman and De Vleesschanwer 1996; Huang and Slevin 1999; Office for National Statistics 2002). The stress of caring may also impact on physical health and stress-related illness such as high blood pressure as well as emotional problems (Weinberg and Huxley 2000; Rethink 2003). On the other hand, they may find themselves marginalized by professionals who may appear to remain indifferent to their situation and fail to provide adequate information and support (Rethink 2003).

The notion of responsibility also has some basis within legislation. A survey of carers' organizations by Berzins (2003) across Europe identified that in one half of all the countries surveyed, relatives had some level of legal involvement in authorizing compulsory detention and that in a minority of countries this was extended to families being held accountable for actions committed by their relative with a mental health problem (Spain) or a legal responsibility on discharge or leave of absence from hospital (Cyprus). In Scotland, the potential for conflict or the breakdown of relationships between user/survivor and family has led to the removal of legislative involvement, whilst in England and Wales new mental health legislation reflects a rethinking of the role of the nearest relative. Previous legislation has been particularly contentious in its rigid definitions of 'family' and has long been criticized for neither corresponding to who has undertaken the caring role nor recognizing user/survivor choice. This was particularly significant when relationships – for example, between lesbian or gay partners – were not recognized and where, in some situations, family members who may have been perpetrators of abuse, were not identified.

In England and Wales, the needs of carers are addressed by the *National Service Framework for Mental Health* (DOH 1999a). Standard 6 supports the provision in the Carers (Recognition and Services) Act (1995) that sets out the requirement that anyone caring for someone subjct to the CPA should have an annual assessment of their own caring, physical and mental health needs and have their own written care plan. This has been backed up by additional funding and additional guidance *Developing Services for Carers and Families of People with Mental Illness* (DOH 2002c). *The NHS Plan* (DOH 2000b) also makes a general commitment to provide additional staff to strengthen carer support networks and increased resources for respite care. As with the earlier Carers (Recognition and Services) Act (1995) and the Carers and Disabled Children Act (2000), which includes the right of carers to an assessment and support, there is as yet little evidence of the systematic and comprehensive implementation of these objectives, although there is some evidence of innovative work and projects in some areas (Rethink 2003).

A further dimension of support for carers of people with mental health difficulties stems from the development of family interventions, based on the notion of expressed emotion, referred to earlier in this chapter. This approach, incorporating information, relapse prevention and the development of problem-solving strategies, is now embedded within guidelines from the National Institute for Clinical Excellence (NICE) (2002). These recommend that family interventions should be routinely offered to all families of people diagnosed as having schizophrenia who are living with or in close contact with service users, and that this should last for a minimum of six months incorporating at least ten sessions. This guidance also needs to be set alongside the increasing numbers of crisis resolution and home treatment teams which are attempting to divert hospital inpatient admissions. Whilst this is generally a desirable objective given the accounts of user/survivor experiences, it is important also to consider the consequences of managing acute periods of ill-health or distress within the home and the impact on carers and family members.

Within the spirit of the NICE guidance, there have also been a number of innovative developments involving carers as trainers, alongside professionals, in projects designed to provide information, support and coping strategies. The Carers Education and Support Programme offered by Rethink is based on a ten-week course co-led by carers and professionals. It aims to increase the knowledge, skills and confidence of the carers of people diagnosed as having severe mental illnesses (Rethink 2004).

With regard to government policy, 'carers' have featured prominently since the early 1990s and their financial importance in terms of saved expenditure on public services has been acknowledged. This is coupled, however, with a tendency to regard 'carers' as a homogenous rather than a heterogeneous grouping and to coalesce the interests of service users and carers. A particular aspect of this concerns the gendered dimension of caring and the need to acknowledge the role of carers from black and minority ethnic communities. Given what has been described as 'the dearth of research on the mental health care experience of minority ethnic groups' (National Institute for Mental Health in England [NIMHE] 2003c), it is perhaps hardly surprising that little is known about the experiences of carers from such groups. The information that is available comes from local reports and voluntary sector groups and projects, supplemented by inquiry findings which point to the inadequate involvement of families and carers in the treatment and care of people from black and minority ethnic communities. A report by Hepworth (2000) identified that for all carers from black and minority ethnic communities, including those caring for people with mental health difficulties, one of the key issues appears to be the need to enable carers to access systems of information and support within mainstream services. There may also be issues of identity whereby certain groups do not perceive themselves as 'carers'. Additional concerns include the availability of culturally sensitive services and information in languages other than English (Arshad and Johal 1999). A consistent message is the need for further research into the needs and experiences of carers from black and minority ethnic groups (Arksey 2002).

The issues concerning women as carers in respect of people with mental health difficulties are in themselves complex and require careful examination. More generally, the history of care as a concept is associated with the differing associations of public and privatized notions of care, underpinned by gendered understandings of the role of women in both paid and unpaid aspects of care, especially in relation to children and older people. Various critiques of care in the community have addressed the assumptions made concerning the role of women as unpaid and unrecognized carers, whilst others have acknowledged women's role in the workforce as poorly paid and of low status. Such critiques have often referred to the stereotypical assumptions of women's responsibilities as carers within and outside the home and the inevitable association with poverty and lack of opportunities for advancement through training and education.

As already indicated it is important to avoid simplistic and dichotomous explanations, whilst also recognizing the limited information available. First it is important to acknowledge that many women who have experience of mental distress themselves will also be carers, either of children or other family members and neighbours, and that these roles are frequently overlooked. Second, women with caring responsibilities are particularly vulnerable to mental ill-health (DOH 2002a) with 40% of women spending over 50 hours a week caring for someone living with them (Corti and Dex 1995). Whilst it is important not to overlook the contribution made by male carers, there are suggestions that for male carers the impact of caring may be ameliorated by a higher level of positive feedback and recognition (Rose and Bruce 1995), and that, in general, men are less subject to gendered expectations of care and caring which are seen to underpin and inform community care (Finch and Groves 1983; Fisher 1997). Wheeler's research into the mental health of black and minority ethnic women (1994) also draws attention to the finding that men tend to be discharged from mental health inpatient services into the care of their wives, whilst women return home to resume the full-time care of their homes and children.

Returning to the tensions and dilemmas referred to earlier in this section it seems important to consider if and how these might be resolved at the level of the lived situations of individuals and their family and friends, recognizing the particular issues as they affect women and black and minority ethnic communities. There is clearly a need for greater availability of and access to information and support and a stronger sense of partnership between carers and professionals. Greater clarity concerning issues of confidentiality and the need to meet the needs of carers in their own right might also go some way towards tackling the complexities of differing interests, needs and priorities without re-enforcing inequality and dependency. As has been suggested elsewhere:

It may be that a good quality service for users is also a good quality service for carers.

(NIMHE 2003c: 4)

MENTAL HEALTH AND CITIZENSHIP

In relation to citizenship, there are many models. Oliver (1996) from within the disability movement has drawn from the work of T H Marshall to equate citizenship with the achievement of political, social and civil rights. He has used these rights as a yardstick to measure 'lack', advocating anti-discrimination legislation as the means to tackle shortfalls to enable disabled people to fully participate in society as citizens. Lister (1997, 2002) views citizenship as a dynamic process which contains elements related to 'status' that incorporates rights and outcomes, and elements related to 'practice' that emphasize process and the right of all to participate as political citizens. Lister ensures that difference and diversity are fully incorporated into understandings of citizenship to avoid citizenship containing exclusionary mechanisms. In this, Lister's approach clearly differs from that of the Labour government where citizenship rights are clearly linked to largely undifferentiated obligations, such as the obligation to support oneself by undertaking paid work. As discussed in Chapter 5, the importance of work is prioritized in Labour's conception of citizenship, leaving those on the margins to struggle in a web of social inclusion initiatives that appear to fall short of full citizenship, or to warrant 'security' and the continuation of the exclusionary care and control measures that this entails.

The Labour government has ensured that employment retains a central position in its social inclusion agenda. However, for users/survivors, the benefits system remains unhelpful. To claim benefit, it is inability not ability that has to be emphasised and this is reinforced by the personal capacity assessment. Similarly, the Incapacity Benefit 'permitted work' rules are so convoluted, that for many the strain of finding out what is possible and what is not and the ongoing danger of being regarded as 'too capable' and/or making a mistake resulting in the loss of some or all entitlement is just too great. Beresford pertinently poses the question: 'How can such a draconian and incomprehensible system be allowed to coexist with government strictures for service users to get involved in policy and provision and to be paid accordingly?' (2003a: 20). He proposes a social model approach with a focus on addressing the barriers to employment together with an integrated employment strategy for mental health service users. This would comprise a simplified and flexible benefits system orientated towards the actual employment needs of users/survivors. It would involve extending the provisions of the Disability Rights Commission and the work it is undertaking to counter job discrimination, the strengthening of the Disability Discrimination Act 1995 in the move towards accessible and supportive workplaces, the further rolling out of direct payments, and real attempts to tackle the overall quality of working conditions, particularly the incidence of stress in the workplace. Perkins (2003) argues that the dichotomy between those who are employable and those deemed 'incapable' or 'invalid' needs to be abolished. She argues that there needs to be a major overhaul of the wages/benefits system, replacing the capable/incapable distinction with a continuum of capacity to work. She advocates something like a simple 50% rule to facilitate ease of movement between work and benefit. Accordingly if a person in receipt of benefit works for an hour he or she could receive 50% of their income with the state offsetting 50% against benefits. She also calls for greater employer flexibility with regard to working hours and for the introduction of annual hours contracts.

Professionals have also contributed towards citizenship debates for those seen to have mental health problems. Huxley and Thornicroft (2004), for example, identify two different meanings for 'social exclusion'. They identify *'demos'* as having implications for citizens' rights, whilst *'ethnos'* has implications for practising clinicians. *Demos* is regarded as relating to those rights conferred by states, with *ethnos* referring to a cultural community with shared values, identification and a sense of cohesion. They see psychiatrists being influential at both levels. With regard to *demos*, for example, psychiatrists can campaign for greater awareness of depression and the stigma attached to mental ill-health. In relation to *ethnos*, psychiatrists can focus on 'social quality' and the interrelationships between minority ethnic culture and mental illness. They assert that psychiatrists need to engage in *demos*-related changes as well as *ethnos*-related measures in order to 'lead to greater social inclusion and a reduction of the stigma of mental illness' (2004: 4).

Bracken and Thomas (2004) advocate a different approach. They make clear links between post-psychiatry, which they insist is not another model, and a form of citizenship which has both active and passive modes. Active modes they define as engaging in political activity as well as defining one's own identity and celebrating this in different ways. Passive modes refer to entitlement to rights and welfare as well as freedom from discrimination, exclusion and oppression. They see active and passive citizenship as being indivisible. They challenge professionals to move beyond the easy fix of the 'diagnose and treat' medical model and to focus on an active citizenship agenda where those areas important to service users – dignity, engagement, trust and regaining hope – determine provision. They assert:

> The citizenship agenda recognizes the importance of better treatments and services. It supports campaigns against discrimination and stigma. But it also works to bind these to increasing demands from user groups for spaces in which some fundamental assumptions about mental health can be questioned.
>
> (Bracken and Thomas 2004: 7)

Bracken and Thomas maintain that mental illness or, in the terms they prefer, 'states of madness, distress or alienation' are social phenomena that require a social response. They recommend a community development approach and stress the principle of mutual support. They strongly advocate moving 'the agenda out of the clinic and into the community' (2004: 13). By doing this, they have importantly taken the concept of citizenship and applied it to psychiatric practice. As a result, debates which have been marginalized within survivor movements are being taken into the mainstream and are making a significant contribution to understandings of citizenship within mental health.

However, with regard to associations between citizenship and the concern of the government to generate social and community capital, users/survivors tend not to feature. The government is keen to generate social capital by building the capacity of local communities. As has often been said, 'community' is a word with many different meanings and communities have the potential to exclude as well as include (Barnes 1997; Pereira 1997). In terms of forging partnerships between community groupings to drive urban regeneration, many authors have drawn attention to such partnerships being far from equal (Atkinson 1999; Power 2001). Users/survivors comprise communities of interest and it is clear that with regard to the production of social capital, these communities continue to be subjected to the exclusionary practices of other communities. Citizenship and inclusion are about social cohesion and emphasizing commonalities rather than differences. This area is explored further in Chapter 8 but it is possible to assert that the government, by continuing to differentiate communities of users/survivors from other communities and to sanction the use of segregatory criteria, can be seen to be perpetuating rather than ameliorating or addressing this process.

CONCLUDING REMARKS

Over recent decades, there can be seen to have been a polarization of thinking about disability and mental health. On both sides, there has been a tendency to privilege particular conceptualizations and only to acknowledge opposing views when these can be seen to fit or made to fit with the prevailing tenets. This can be seen within psychiatry and the pharmaceutical industry as well as within the disability movement. There is clearly a need to move beyond an individual, pathologizing approach into one that emphasizes how disability is socially constructed and to acknowledge the implication and effect of power imbalances. This is not to argue for the replacement of one monolith by another. It is important for social model tenets to be used to inform understandings and construct challenges, but any rigidity of application would prevent rather than facilitate the goals of choice, the celebration of difference and the exercise of autonomy. In relation to psychiatry, the work of Bracken and Thomas, Fernando, Shashidaran and others heralds important changes. Tensions will and indeed should remain, but it is also clear that the dynamics of the debate are shifting and the importance of this cannot be overemphasized.

7 Experts and allies – workers, professionals, service users and carers

> There are no experts in misery or madness, only experts at claiming expertise.
>
> (Pilgrim 1998: 23)

This chapter sets out to explore issues concerning all the players involved in the delivery of mental health services and to identify some of the current trends and tensions which may be present, including the involvement of service users and survivors as well as the shift towards multi-agency and interprofessional working. Whilst a range of occupations – for example, nursing – have historically been concerned with the care of people with mental health difficulties, the picture is rapidly changing. At one level there is an increasing number of professional groups shuffling for position in various multi-disciplinary and multi-agency settings, whilst at another, new occupational categories are being created and extended, such as support workers and the recently established *Support, Time and Recovery (STR) Workers* in England (DOH 2003b). A critical development concerns the significance of the increasing involvement of users and carers not only as active participants in service development and evaluation but also as employed members of mental health teams (Perkins and Repper 1999; Carling and Allott 1999). Notwithstanding this, to some extent, there have always been and continue to be, members of the workforce who have experienced their own mental health difficulties but have not felt confident in declaring this publicly.

All of these territories – that is, those of the various disciplines and the service users – are now being contested and challenged from a number of different directions within a rapidly changing external environment. This wider picture includes the changing organizational context of health and social care services and the shifting patterns of workforce configurations, influenced by the drive towards occupational standards and competence frameworks with an emphasis on a flexible and multi-skilled workforce (DOH 2000a; SCMH 2000). The increasing introduction of non-professionally aligned support workers, that is, those without professional qualifications, in a variety of posts and settings will also be considered within what may be seen as a move towards 'deprofessionalization', which also recognizes the value placed on such workers by service users and carers (SCMH 1997; Burns et al 2001).

At a wider level, concepts of modernity and postmodernity may be relevant to assist in the exploration of the changing understandings of the roles of health and social care professionals. Psychiatry, alongside psychology and sociology, is clearly associated with modernity and the quest for knowledge. Medical discourse on 'illness', 'disease' and 'disability' has contributed towards an overall 'objectification' process by which illness has concentrated on viewing in isolation from people as individuals. Bury refers to the key processes of objectification, rationalization and subjectification which characterize the shift from modernity to postmodernity in relation to illness and health and medicine (1998: 24).

> To fall ill meant to call in the doctor, increasingly meaning someone working within the confines of a regulated professional organization and someone working with a scientific view of disease.
>
> (Bury 1998: 7)

This shift can also be seen as a means by which it is only the doctor, as a professional, who:

> . . . can know the truth about illness through the language of disease, and the patient becomes a passive agent.
>
> (Ibid)

At the beginning of the twenty-first century, it is possible to identify an apparent shift away from the power relationships between professional and 'patient' exemplified above. This has been influenced by, for example, the increasing availability of knowledge and information, a cynicism towards the traditional belief that 'doctors know best' and a growing and increasingly legitimized interest in alternative and complementary approaches to health and health care. Paradoxically, however, it is also possible to see how concepts from medicine in general and psychiatry in particular, as well as from the other social sciences, including sociology and psychology, are being extended from the realm of illness into the social world where increasingly they are contributing to systems of surveillance. Armstrong (1995) highlights the role of 'surveillance medicine' whereby extensive information concerning individuals and groups is collected and analysed and the maintenance of a healthy life-style, both physically and emotionally, is held to be the responsibility of informed 'consumers'. Ostensibly underpinned by notions of choice and free will, these factors may also be questionable if the concept of governmentality is considered which, it is suggested, concerns both coercive and non-coercive strategies that may be utilized to ensure that individuals take the responsibility allocated to them. Examples of this might include the role of insurance companies in accessing health information when considering life assurance and the use of sensitive information concerning family history or sexual behaviours.

The shift from objectification to subjectification, associated with the shift towards postmodernity, is understood by some to bring its own risks as there is increasing emphasis on exploring and explaining our own emotional and psychological well-being, paradoxically accepting responsibility and taking heed of guidance from an increasing range of 'experts'. In offering their services in response to all aspects of the human condition – for example, in response to bereavement, anxiety and stress – such experts thereby also extend their professional remit, rendering such subjective experience as central to their task. From yet another perspective, however, it is also possible to see that it is the process of subjectification which can also be regarded as creating possibilities for the voices of marginalized groups to be heard, including women, black and minority ethnic groups and those with experience of mental distress.

There are conflicting views about the injection of emotions and subjectivity into the social world. At one level there is an increasing trend towards eliciting personal accounts and stories by listening to the voices of those who have experienced distress and those who have used services but alternatively authenticity may be regarded as illusory. Attempts at resisting care or specific interventions can be seen as denial and ultimately the scope of counselling and therapy is extended into every area of life.

> Signs of resistance are recycled by the practitioner as a concern for the patient's emotional and subjective well-being.
>
> (Bury 1998: 16)

This chapter will begin by taking an historical perspective across the various professional groups involved in mental health care, including psychiatry, nursing and social work, taking into account the development of the respective roles and the boundaries between the various components of the workforce. The implications of these roles for relationships between workers and those with whom they are working will also be explored to consider the ways in which traditional boundaries have been drawn and maintained and the purpose and implications of what has historically been a clear-cut distinction.

The chapter will raise a number of questions concerning the future of the mental health workforce including who is best equipped to deliver the range of services and interventions which are seen to be required. What future is there for the traditional professional roles and are current developments paving the way for the introduction of a generic mental health worker? A crucial question concerns the pivotal position of service users and carers and the complex power issues which are associated with moves towards increasing involvement at a number of levels within the system.

Issues of language have already been raised in Chapters 1 and 6 concerning the use of such terms as 'service users', 'people with mental health difficulties' and 'survivors'. It may, however, be appropriate here to consider the language and concepts associated with the term 'professional'. For example, a clear line is frequently drawn between professional and non-professional workers, a distinction that re-enforces the hierarchical distinction between those who hold a professional qualification and those who do not. The concept of 'professional' also implicitly brings into being the concept of 'client' or 'patient', representing an example of a binary distinction. Such binary or dichotomous concepts are frequently represented as oppositional thinking in terms of either one category or another, such as the notion of black or white, male or female, or, as in this instance, professional or client/patient, thereby leading to only a partial and incomplete consideration of complex issues. As Fook (2002) suggests, this limits the recognition and understanding of complex identities and implies that categories are mutually exclusive, as is the case with the example given.

The term 'professional' has a range of meanings, each of which carries its own shades and nuances. Overall, however, it can be seen as a 'discourse' that conveys a particular set of ideas and beliefs, which, as such, can be critically examined or deconstructed in order to reveal underlying power relationships. Conventional features of 'professional' include the possession of certain attributes: work for remuneration; public trust; professional neutrality; practice underpinned by knowledge base; a long period of training creating a close-knit 'community'; and a code of ethics creating professional autonomy. Traditional notions of professional life have been summarized by Carrier and Kendall (1995) as offering:

> . . . a claim to sapiential authority, high ethical standards and autonomy based upon the judicious use of discretion and judgement on behalf of clients.
>
> (Carrier and Kendall 1995: 11)

As they go on to explore an alternative perspective, it is clear that such a definition is open to challenge at a number of levels. Whilst accountability and responsibility would seem to be intrinsic elements of what it means to be a professional, recent years have seen a number of examples where such assumptions have been undermined and suspicions raised concerning the behaviour of professionals. This would include, for example, inquiries into the use of human organs (Redfern 2001), the behaviour of individual practitioners (Smith 2002), and aspects of institutional abuse within institutional care (Fallon 1999). Such inquiries have articulated a growing concern that neither individual practitioners nor organizations and institutions conform with public expectations of accountability and transparency and confirm a widely held view that:

The very existence of occupations which make claims to expertise in areas of health and welfare may be said to have been founded on the exclusion of users from the definition of need or appropriate responses to its remedy.

(Hugman 1998: 137)

Such experiences and many others might suggest that notions of 'profession' are located within systems of power and status, and as such are of benefit to the professional rather than the client, offering a means of protection through processes of social exclusion and gatekeeping, often associated with inequalities in terms of gender, race and class. Furthermore claims for expertise and knowledge may be uncertain and open to challenge. Again specific examples can be identified to support this critique in respect of mental health and examples of Eurocentric and male bias within the development of psychiatry will be examined further.

This chapter will now consider the various ways in which 'professional expertise' is being challenged within mental health services and, in so doing, will highlight issues of power and inequality. First it will be necessary to locate the evidence within the wider political and social context in which there has been an increasing trend towards the reduction of the power base hitherto held by professionals. This will include the effects of the growing trend towards interprofessional and multi-agency working and the increasing flexibility demanded of workers operating in teams regardless of their professional background. Second, the growth of the mental health workforce and increasing demands for workers will be considered in terms of the impact on the service. This will include organizational and professional aspects as well as issues concerning the quality and purpose of the service and the related training and educational requirements. The third dimension of this analysis will consider relationships with service users and carers, including their involvement and participation in service delivery at a number of levels, building on the issues already raised in Chapter 6. Finally a number of key themes will be drawn together in an attempt to make sense of a number of contradictions and challenges.

TRADITIONAL PROFESSIONAL ROLES

The development of psychiatry as a medical specialism has already been referred to in the wider historical development of mental health policy and practice and its continuing dominance has been described by various commentators (Treacher and Baruch, 1980; Bracken and Thomas 2001; Double 2002a). For our purposes here, issues concerning race, gender and psychiatry and the role of psychiatry alongside other professions will be considered, together with the response of the psychiatric profession to the challenge of changing expectations and policy imperatives.

In considering the impact of psychiatry and its emergence within a particular historical context, the origins of present-day concerns regarding oppressive and discriminatory practice can be found in nineteenth-century and early twentieth-century psychiatry. Fernando (2002) points to how psychiatry developed as a profession at a particular historical period. As this period was associated with the rise of scientific racism, it resulted in the embedding of Eurocentric and racist attitudes at the heart of psychiatric knowledge with regard to diagnosis and treatment. Such developments were preceded by the move towards a disease model as opposed to a reliance on religious concepts and understandings and the notion of the mind and the 'mental physiology' of the brain as a parallel to that of the body. These in turn gave rise to complex classificatory systems based on a hierarchy of illness and single factor causation. Psychiatry was also associated with social Darwinism and the view that races were at different stages of development and the eugenics movement, which sought to identify and then eradicate 'inferior' races. Rousseau's concept of the 'noble savage' untainted by Western civilization and free from insanity (or mental degeneracy as the lack of Western culture and the allegation that freedom as opposed to slavery was regarded as the cause of madness), also provides an insight into such thinking. There is, however, more recent evidence that racist thinking continues to permeate psychiatric knowledge and practices including, for example, the debate concerning the higher incidence of schizophrenia amongst the African-Caribbean population in Britain and the higher rates of detention under the mental health legislation, which has been referred to in Chapter 4.

The picture concerning psychiatry and views of women, again as seen in Chapter 4, offers a rather similar picture in terms of the underpinning knowledge base, interpretations of thinking and behaviour and associated practices. The experiences of women have been well analysed and documented both from a historical perspective (e.g. Chesler 1972; Showalter 1987) and in terms of more recent policy and practice (Payne 1998; Busfield 2001) and the impact of the experiences of inequality, discrimination and disadvantage can be seen to operate at the level of women's day-to-day experiences as well as their treatment within mental health services.

As increasing understanding of complex processes developed further, the emergence of multi-factorial models to explain the aetiology of mental illness, including psychological and social approaches, has led to the notion of eclecticism. Rather than representing a serious challenge to the conceptual pre-ordinance of the medical model and the crucial role of disease processes underpinning traditional psychiatry, Goldie suggests that the absorption, rather than the rejection, of new ideas has enabled psychiatry to retain its hold on the diagnosis and treatment of mental illness. In referring to Goldie's work, Treacher and Baruch (1980) argue that this strategy is one of many in a continuing process of maintaining medical hegemony in this field, citing the move to locate psychiatric care within district general hospitals celebrated in the 1971 White Paper, *Hospital Services for the Mentally Ill* (Department of Health and Social Security [DHSS] 1971).

Nursing, whilst drawing heavily on the conceptual and theoretical frameworks offered from within medicine, and sometimes perceived to undertake a 'handmaiden' role with all of the associated gendered interpretations, can also be seen as having a complex trajectory in terms of its development as a profession. In his discussion of the development of mental health nursing, Nolan comments that:

> Having a history confirms the legitimacy of the service one provides: mere inclusion in the history of another group implies mere subordination.
>
> (Nolan 1993: 1)

The historical development of mental health nursing as a specialism can also be charted via the attendants and 'keepers' of the asylums, the mental nurses and psychiatric nurses and what has been described as a continuing 'quest for a unique role' (Nolan 1993: 13). In many respects this also concerns an ambivalent relationship with both medicine and general nursing as well as with psychiatry which can be traced in the changes over the years to the training and education of nurses. These include the changing content of courses ranging from biological sciences, an emphasis on interpersonal relationships (Peplau 1952), approaches grounded in skills development, and increasing attention being paid to social sciences. Additionally, the changing relationship with general nursing mirrors wider twists and turns, from entirely separate training located in psychiatric hospitals to the shared common foundation programme based within academic institutions for all would-be nurses, regardless of their intended area of work.

The development of nursing in relation to the care of people with mental health problems can also be seen as being characterized as shifting between an instrumental and task-focused approach and a pastoral, therapeutic role. In relation to nursing education, this is represented as a clinical emphasis on physical care as compared to patient-centred nursing where the pastoral role of the nurse and associated emotional work becomes central to the nursing process. With regard to mental health, this can be seen in the contrast between the role of the nurse in administering medication, and that of the nurse as therapist, where the relationship is paramount.

In many ways both social work and occupational therapy have, not unlike nursing, been characterized as quasi-professions. Both of the former groups have historically developed at a greater distance from the overall surveillance of the medical profession whilst, conversely, both social work and occupational therapy have also maintained the notion of a generic professional identity not confined to any one area of work.

In England, specific training for social workers in mental health commenced in 1929 at the London School of Economics (Timms 1964: 21) following interest in similar developments in the USA. In the same year and again influenced by a visit to the USA Dr Elizabeth Casson set up the first school of occupational therapy at Dorset House in Bristol. Encouraged by a recommendation from the Board of Control (set up by the Royal Commission for the Care of the Feeble-minded, 1904–8, with responsibilities for comprehensive services for the insane, senile, epileptic, feeble-minded, idiots and imbeciles), the intention was to develop an almoner-type role responsible for allaying patients' anxieties about home during treatment and helping with employment and domestic issues after discharge from hospital. The key to occupational therapy rested on the need to pay attention to both mental motivation and physical experience.

By 1950 only 523 students had qualified as psychiatric social workers with only a small minority employed by local authority mental welfare departments. Instead departments were staffed by duly authorized relieving officers and workers from voluntary associations (Jones 1972; Timms 1964). Those trained as psychiatric social workers were largely employed within mental health services including child guidance and the voluntary sector organizations and remained separate from local government departments. This was accentuated by the specialized nature of the early training which emphasized work with people with serious emotional disturbance rather than a wider form of social casework (Younghusband 1964; Seed 1973).

The 1959 Mental Health Act introduced the role of the mental welfare officer, which then became the approved social worker (ASW) in the 1983 legislation. The purpose of these roles was to offer a lay perspective to the process of assessment for compulsory admission to hospital. On the one hand this development served to strengthen the base for mental health social work within local authority departments, although the recommendations of the Seebohm Report in 1968, for the replacement of various specialisms in terms of child care, the welfare of older people and mental health, including learning disability, by one generic social worker, could be viewed as potentially reversing this process. Within the new generic social services departments child care and child protection were established as the over-riding priority and apart from the statutory work required by legislation, mental health work remained the province of unqualified workers who dealt primarily with the remainder. The lack of attention to mental health, as well as the caution with which many social workers viewed mainstream psychiatry, has been seen as a factor in the increasing development of the role of the community psychiatric nurse (CPN). The CPN has been able to take on the role of supporting people in the community after discharge with the added benefits of being able to administer medication as well as a familiarity with and an acceptance of the medical model and traditional hierarchical relationships within psychiatry.

In many respects all the groups identified so far can be seen to be constantly negotiating and renegotiating their roles and tasks along a continuum which moves between an emphasis on task and an emphasis on relationship. Whilst many would suggest that the latter orientation sits more comfortably alongside an individual's search for meaning within a user-determined definition of recovery, this increasing concern with the whole world of the individual may be experienced as intrusive and one where any attempt at resistance is construed as denial, within which interpretation, once again, the expert knows best.

Psychology both as a subject discipline underpinning counselling and wide-ranging forms of therapy and as the profession of clinical psychology could be seen as also having to contend with the need to challenge the historical role of 'handmaiden' to a medically driven approach to mental health. However, to some extent psychology has also demonstrated the possibility of resistance from an independent perspective with the benefits of a recognized knowledge base, lengthy training and its own attempt to claim territorial ownership of certain aspects of mental health work, particularly those concerned with psychoanalytic and behavioural approaches. The move towards direct referral from GPs to clinical psychology services introduced by the Trethowan Report (DHSS 1977), also widened the gap with psychiatry. More recently the increasing involvement of psychological approaches to working with psychosis based on cognitive behavioural therapy has similarly reinforced the distinctiveness of psychology. The British Psychological Society (2000) has endorsed psychology's contribution to the field, although the actual numbers of psychologists, *vis-à-vis* nurses and social workers, remains small.

It is evident that the contribution of different professional groups to mental health services remains dynamic and contested and, in turning our attention towards the contemporary picture of multi-disciplinary team working as a key feature of current developments, it is important to consider how these historical trends and tensions are being managed.

One feature of the contemporary scene is the role of psychiatry and the extent to which this remains the central linchpin of service organization and delivery. Whilst some might point to the declining role of psychiatry within mental health services, or at least to a shift in overall dominance as a result of growing interest in social or multi-factorial models of mental distress or illness, there are indications that despite the influence of the post-psychiatry movement, the close alliance of psychiatry and biomedicine is being maintained and extended. Advances in knowledge in neuroscience and genetics maintain the potential dominance of biological and medical approaches within a neo-Kraepelinian model, whilst critics of psychiatry's extending role, outside of the traditional domain, point to the increasing involvement in the social and political arena and the medicalization of everyday problems (Double 2002a).

In support of this argument Double (2002a) points to the increase in the diagnosis of attention deficit hyperactivity disorder in children and the overlap with the kinds of behaviour associated with boredom or stress.

There is also the medical reframing of shyness as a social anxiety disorder and the development of the diagnosis of post-traumatic stress disorder as a human response to disaster or trauma to consider.

There is also an increasing recognition that psychiatrists are overburdened and that their role is confusing, complex, and rapidly changing. They are expected to provide leadership, management and accountability, a range of clinical expertise and care co-ordination. At the same time it has been acknowledged that:

> Much power stems from doctors' relationship to the social institution of illness. In arbitrating and administering this doctors define changes in the rights and responsibilities of patients, society and those around them. This institution is an integral part of the functioning of society as a whole . . .
>
> (National Working Group on New Roles for Psychiatrists 2004: 13)

The development of the role of the CPN has been seen as creating the opportunity for mental health nursing to develop outside the hospital and away from close supervision by the medical profession. The terminology appears to be moving away from psychiatric to mental health nursing, possibly marking a move away from psychiatry/medicine towards a wider and more holistic approach to mental health. Mental health nurses are now found to be key members of a range of community teams including community mental health teams, assertive outreach, crisis resolution and home treatment teams and often operate as team leaders and clinical managers within such settings. These developments mark an increasing trend towards mental health nurses operating independently of consultant psychiatrists and often accepting referrals directly from GPs in primary care.

Despite being located within multi-disciplinary teams, many mental health social workers continue to remain employed by local authority social services departments and may find themselves party to conflicting loyalties and pressures. Often they remain firmly embedded in a psychiatric social work team with a corresponding set of legislative allegiances and duties. At the same time they are also likely to belong to a multi-disciplinary team where their presence, salience and involvement on a day-to-day basis may be limited by other demands. In practice the role may swing between providing a supporting role to the health care team, frequently characterized as offering housing or benefits advice, to a more broadly therapeutic role with individuals and their families that has much in common with those of other professionals. At times social workers may also feel responsible for maintaining a minority position upholding a social perspective in the face of the overwhelming presence of the medical model, whilst at other times they may be faced with a sense that the collective ownership of a social model by other members of the team renders them redundant.

The sense of redundancy has also been exacerbated by the new mental health legislation, whereby the role of the ASW has been replaced by that of the approved mental health professionals, from any one of a number of professional backgrounds. At a time when the future of local authority social services departments is increasingly uncertain, the development of children's trusts, care trusts and joint mental health trusts (to be discussed further elsewhere) suggests a number of future scenarios for mental health social work, not all of which may be viewed positively.

There are also concerns regarding the wider understanding of the role of occupational therapists within community mental health services and inter-professional rivalries which continue to threaten the availability of an appropriate service (Onyett et al 1994). There is evidence of a growing emphasis on the development of collaborative and partnership initiatives as part of the combined undertakings of the College of Occupational Therapists and the Royal College of Psychiatrists (2002). This is endorsed by the report of the SCMH (1997) which also refers to the need for the training of occupational therapists to focus on the management of severe mental illness within the community setting, as well as to prepare for new roles within primary health care. Again, numbers are small, and whilst figures from 1998 (Craik et al 1998) indicate that there were 23,000 state-registered occupational therapists in the UK, only 30% are to be found in mental health.

The configuration of mental health services, considered further elsewhere, also plays a part in the shifting roles between the various occupational groups. Interprofessional working, whilst frequently claimed or exhorted, may be variously demonstrated across primary care, inpatient and commu-nity-based services as well as in non-statutory services. The much-used phrase 'multi-professional team working' frequently conceals as much as it reveals and is fundamentally influenced by factors such as team structure, management and lines of accountability, as well as by the extent to which a shared ethos, approach and knowledge base exists. That is not to suggest that different and, at times, contesting views, may not be held, but that there is a need for a transparent decision-making process and that team working arrangements should be founded on recognition and respect for ideological differences (Colombo et al). In reality, despite the rhetoric, many teams demonstrate continuing parallel and uniprofessional perspectives, leading Onyett (2003) when reviewing the evidence for the effectiveness of team working, to conclude that team effectiveness cannot be assumed.

Understandings of 'professional' also need to be seen in the wider chang-ing context of health and social care. The increasing permeation of the values and language of the market place, highlighted by the NHS and Community Care Act 1990, has led to terms such as 'patient' or 'client' transmogrifying into those of 'consumer' or 'service user'. Whilst at one level this terminology suggests an increased concern with rights and choices, at another the terms obscure issues of scarce resources and rationing and the continuation of inequalities within the decision-making process. Consumerism is also associated with the shift from modernity to postmodernity. Here, as Bury (1998) points out, competition and customer service, where 'choice' and 'preference' re-enforce notions of subjectivity, have the potential to open up possibilities of complementary and holistic medicine (1998: 4).

Increasing regulation of the process of training and registration has been associated with a growing emphasis on models of competence, performance indicators and the gathering of evidence to demonstrate skills in practice. Whilst the requirement to demonstrate competence can only be advantageous for practice, there is a risk that a preoccupation with detailed checklists of performance indicators may lead to a reductionist emphasis on complying with protocol and procedures and losing sight of the subtleties required for a more holistic and responsive approach to complex human situations. This is particularly the case for mental health where there is a need to understand the uniqueness of each individual and her or his circumstances.

In respect of mental health services, the current 'modernization' agenda is rapidly moving forward in terms of education and training for the mental health workforce, driven by the *National Service Framework for Mental Health* (DOH 1999a) and developments concerning the wider context of health and social care services. *A Health Service for All the Talents* (DOH 2000a) emphasizes the need for a flexible and multi-skilled workforce and this is reflected in the Mental Health Workforce Action Team report (DOH 2000b) stressing the importance of inter-disciplinary and inter-agency education and training and the need for collaborative working, recognizing the increased 'blurring' of professional roles. The report states that:

> Increasingly workforce planning will be based around the competences required to deliver services rather than around numbers of professional staff.
>
> (DOH 2000b: 41)

The process is being furthered through the introduction of core occupational standards and training for mental health practitioners, which increasingly specifies flexible roles and the transfer of skills and knowledge across hitherto clear-cut demarcations. Accordingly, an integrated framework, incorporating the occupational standards for mental health, shared capabilities and the knowledge and skills framework, is being constructed building on the concept of *The Capable Practitioner* (SCMH 2000).

A significant development has been a massive increase in the number of those workers described as professionally non-affiliated. Figures suggest that there are in the region of 11,000 mental health support workers who are mostly unqualified and located in day centres, residential homes, community teams and drop-in centres (Improvement and Development Agency 1999). Many are undertaking work formerly within the domain of qualified professionals including taking on assessment and care management tasks under the umbrella of 'support'. Whilst, on the one hand, many busy teams appear to value the contribution of their support worker colleagues, there may be occasions when professional groups have felt undermined by the introduction of less well-qualified and lower-paid colleagues to undertake similar work.

From the point of view of service users the contribution offered by support workers is highly regarded and appreciated for its flexibility and availability (Burns et al 2001). It could also be argued that the role of support workers is embedded in natural and informal support networks and to some extent resembles the level of care and support that would otherwise be offered by friends and family. There is good reason to believe, however, that the skill and experience of support workers surpass those of concerned friends and relatives (SCMH 1997). A further factor is that support workers may find themselves working independently of professionally qualified staff in many teams and agencies outside of the NHS in social services and voluntary sector services.

Adequate and appropriate training for this group is only now beginning to be offered reflecting a general lack of recognition of the skills and values required and frequently demonstrated by these workers who offer a vital front-line role in providing support and assistance to people with mental health problems living in the community. One explanation for the shortage of training available may be the implicit assumption that these skills are natural and represent everyday demonstrations of common-sense behaviour, possibly linked to gendered expectations of care and carers. In this respect mental health support workers find themselves in a similar position to that of residential workers in social care and other such groups. Another reason can be linked to the view that support workers ought to operate under the guidance of professionals in carrying out predetermined tasks. Overall, support workers are a relatively new phenomenon, linked to the rise of 'community care', and their needs are only now beginning to be recognized and articulated in the training and education arena. There is also an imperative to meet fundamental health and safety requirements as the inquiry into the death of Jonathan Newby in 1993 illustrated (Davies et al 1995).

The increasing role of support workers, however, does raise questions about an agenda of de-professionalization although concerns have not reached the level demonstrated, for example, by teachers' resistance to an increasing role for classroom assistants. Paradoxically, there are also concerns about the quasi-'professionalization' of this group as training and qualification are introduced, detracting from their ability to support people in terms of everyday lives and activities.

For those 'unqualified' or non-professionally affiliated workers committed to a future career in mental health there is no logical progression outside the boundaries of the traditional 'professional' pathways, which paradoxically, in the case of social work and occupational therapy, do not always provide in-depth mental health knowledge and skills at qualifying/registration level. In terms of career development and progression there may be a definite ceiling on the aspirations of support workers however skilled and experienced they may be. There may also be a legitimate concern that the support workers may be drawn from black and minority ethnic groups bringing a much-needed cultural and linguistic sensitivity to mainstream services, but who are then not encouraged to further their own development and potential.

One interpretation of these changes is the suggestion that a new generic mental health worker is the intended outcome, although this is expressly denied in *The Capable Practitioner* (SCMH 2000) which is careful to point out that the description of capabilities across the entire mental health workforce is not an attempt to promote the development of a generic worker. However, the development of mental health support workers would appear inevitably to raise complex questions about professional roles and boundaries. The very term 'non-professionally qualified' in itself attempts to set a clear marker between different groups of workers which in reality may be far muddier and complex than has been fully admitted. At the same time, despite the rhetoric of inter-professional and multi-agency working and the likelihood of care trusts and mental health trusts incorporating health and social care services, and to some extent maybe as a result of it, professionals are continuing to guard their roles and boundaries against forays from other groups, both qualified and unqualified.

An overriding theme of mental health policy concerns the central importance of service user and carer involvement in services at all levels of delivery and, for many with experience of using services over a number of years, the expectation that they will actively participate in decisions concerning their own care and service planning and delivery This represents a significant shift. Indeed, Onyett suggests that: 'It is perhaps more productive to think of the service user as the central team member and to design the rest of the team around them' (2003: 56).

There are a number of complex issues associated with service user and carer involvement. In particular, the utilization of concepts of power and empowerment, and the currency associated with service user experience and its recognition and support, carries with it clear dangers of tokenism and exploitation. One aspect of this concerns the growing employment of people with experience of using services. Whilst this has the potential to fundamentally influence the future development and delivery of services and is to be welcomed, there may be important issues to consider. So far it does not appear that such developments have led to the widespread recruitment of people with user/survivor experience to professional training courses, without which opportunities for progression and promotion will be severely hindered and inequalities maintained. Second, there is a risk that opportunities for employment outwith the mental health services will be overlooked, leaving few choices for anyone who would prefer to seek employment elsewhere. Finally and importantly, there are vital issues relating to equality and the inclusion and integration of service user workers into mental health teams. Despite this, however, the potential benefits are considerable in terms of the quality of support that may be offered by people who have lived experience of mental health difficulties.

CONCLUDING REMARKS

It is apparent that there is a real need for new models of working together, both between the various groups involved in delivering services and in breaking down continuing barriers between those 'providing' and those 'receiving' care. There is much to suggest that new patterns are already evolving and that there are examples of effective team work and positive initiatives in collaborating with users/survivors and carers. However, as yet such developments remain patchy and piecemeal and as a recent report suggests, individuals who use services and their families continue to report not being listened to, being marginal to assessment and care planning and being rendered helpless rather than helped by service use (NIMHE/SCMH/ Joint Workforce Support Unit 2004).

There may also be a sense that it is the overriding importance of values and a commitment to work as allies in the process of recovery that needs to underpin the approach of all those involved in the delivery of mental health services. This might also entail moving away from the traditional role of what Perkins (2004) has described as the 'guilds' who have traditionally held sway, the rethinking of historic roles to ensure their relevance to what service users require and the increasing involvement of new players bringing creative and practical skills as well as the personal experience of mental health problems. An essential aspect of such a development would also require the recognition that all knowledge and experience have a part to play.

8 Change, collaboration and multi-agency working

> Poverty, racism, unemployment, loneliness, relationship difficulties, spiritual conflicts, sexual abuse and domestic violence are at the heart of mental health crises. These phenomena occur within, and are shaped by, different cultural orientations to the world and to suffering and healing. Pills or therapy cannot resolve suffering, and may only make matters worse by obscuring the real reason for distress and alienation.
>
> (Bracken and Thomas 2004: 13)

The intention of this chapter is to consider the complex arrangements which provide a framework for the provision and delivery of mental health services, illustrating the tensions and also the dynamic factors which operate between theory and understandings about mental health, the policy framework and the reality of people's experiences. Within this approach various perspectives are explored to identify a range of possible scenarios for the future, recognizing the common threads or themes which may be present.

Change is a key theme of this chapter, including 'cultural' change in terms of how people understand the experience of mental distress, organizational change relating to the structures which shape the responses to mental health needs, and individual change both within and outwith the frameworks of provision which either exist now or may emerge in the future. The process of change is considered and reviewed as it impacts on various aspects of contemporary mental health, moving through the changing structures and frameworks in both the statutory and voluntary sectors, including the current emphasis on working together.

At a strategic level, key themes are used to consider the shape of services both nationally and regionally in response to government policy and local considerations. Examples of innovative developments are analysed in terms of the stakeholders, associated outcomes and the relationship with the wider picture. Within this wider picture, mental health issues and developments are located within the context of public health and community development initiatives. An important factor is to acknowledge the range of possible agencies that may be involved, including health and social care across the statutory and voluntary sectors, and the level of integration and partnership both within these groups and across the boundary that exists between mental health and other aspects of health and social care in its widest form. For example, this may include reference to community development and broad programmes to tackle inequality and social exclusion. The nature and extent of partnership and joined-up working is also an important consideration.

In particular, the impact and key significance of the public involvement agenda is examined and the extent to which the level of participation of those with experience of using services has been strengthened by this development is explored. Specific perspectives on this debate are appraised with regard to issues of gender and ethnicity and the interrelationship with disadvantage and poverty as part of the overall approach is examined. Returning to the theme of change, the extent to which this represents an overarching realignment of discourses, power and practice is questioned and some of the risks associated with new strategies are appraised.

PROCESS OF CHANGE

The current agenda in the field of mental health,[1] as we have seen, is billed as a 'modernizing' one. This implies that we continue to inhabit a world where 'modern' tenets relating to a continuing commitment to traditional scientific rationality, linear progression, the possibility of a clear diagnosis–treatment continuum and an adherence to expert–patient relationships, retain legitimating authority. However, the presence of clear tensions together with increased fragmentation and diversity can be seen to have contributed to an environment where emphasis has to be placed upon complexity, context and negotiation and the continual evaluation of services to proactively inform policy and practice and to provide a justification for the continuation of support and funding.

As already noted, the process of change in relation to policy, across the wide spectrum of health and social care of which mental health is just one part, is both complex and dynamic, relating to political, organizational and professional imperatives as well as to notions of expressed 'need' and how these can best be addressed. Inevitably the outcomes represent compromise between stakeholders, rather than an orderly sequence of events with a clear underpinning rationale, and may result from unexpected alliances and associations. One example was the wide-ranging opposition to the government's proposals to reform the 1983 Mental Health Act in England. The White Paper published in 2000 brought together the Royal College of Psychiatrists alongside other professional groups and a diverse selection of organizations representing service users and others with personal experience of mental health difficulties (DOH 2000d).

---

1 'Mental health' is the term used in this chapter because it corresponds to the current policy context.

Similarly, at the level of any one organization, change will represent the complex interaction of directives from central government, the internal dynamics of the organization and external drivers concerning local agendas and stakeholder views. Attempts to rationalize this process, drawing on management and business models of change, may all too often founder and not realize the original objectives in terms of improved health outcomes or greater efficiency. The management of change, particularly in response to centrally driven policies, may also not be attainable within the strict time limits imposed to meet political objectives, may lack sufficient resources to ensure rapid delivery or may require significantly longer time to achieve the cultural and local changes and commitment required to underpin the required transformation. For example, the implementation of certain aspects of *The NHS Plan* (DOH 2000b), such as an increase in the numbers of professional staff, although potentially non-contentious, will take many years to achieve given the inevitable time-lag between recruitment and the completion of training and education. More complicated still are government public health objectives such as targets to reduce smoking, increase breast-feeding or cut teenage pregnancies. These all require more than a straightforward change in behaviour and generate debates and pose dilemmas concerning the relative merits or otherwise of strategies designed to impact on individuals, communities and organizations and the advantages of incentives or sanctions to achieve the desired results. Furthermore such debates take place within a political arena where notions of choice and individual responsibility versus government directives and interventions hold sway.

There are numerous examples of frameworks to understand types of organizational change. Amongst the myriad of models available, Ackerman (1997) identifies three types to include developmental, transitional and transformational change, whilst the Audit Commission (2001) identifies four approaches including surgical change, incremental operational gains, evolutionary learning and transformational change. Each of these models is recognized as having benefits and disadvantages, but transformational change is identified as being appropriate to bring about a significant shift in an uncertain environment requiring clear leadership and vision. This also represents radical or second order change and demonstrates marked movement in fundamental processes and assumptions compared to first order change which is demonstrated in alterations and modifications to the existing status quo. Furthermore, in an acknowledgement of the complexity of the process, the Audit Commission report also emphasizes that change must be 'bespoke tailored' and stresses that:

> Change cannot be driven from the centre alone. The government must give local service providers the flexibility to respond to local demands.

Additionally:

> . . . successful change programmes must begin and end with an under-
> standing of what matters to users.
>
> (Audit Commission 2001: 4)

Ideas concerning change and questions concerning the tensions between the
'push' and 'pull' factors designed to effect change and the importance of
winning 'hearts and minds' alongside the need to meet specific targets and
time-scales, will provide an important benchmark for this chapter as it
moves on to explore the current frameworks for the delivery of mental
health services as well as the broader environment within which wider
mental health issues are located and understood.

CHANGE IN STRUCTURES/HEALTH AND SOCIAL CARE/STATUTORY AND VOLUNTARY SECTOR ORGANIZATIONS/PARTNERSHIPS AND JOINED-UP WORKING

Within both mental health services in Britain and the wider framework of
health and social care, key aspects of change concern the imperatives for
working in partnership and 'joined-up working'. In moving to consider
some of the issues associated with this trend, there are a number of
questions which are important to consider. These include the extent to
which this is a transitory development or whether it represents a more
fundamental shift in thinking; the extent to which it reflects and/or
promotes changes in thinking about the nature of mental health difficulties
(for example, the acceptance of a social perspective and a multifactorial
model); and the extent to which it is representative of fundamental transformational change or simply a rewriting of existing ways of thinking about
and providing services illustrative of first order rather than second order
change.

In order to understand partnership developments in mental health it is
helpful to consider the wider context for collaborative developments
stemming back to the inauguration of the NHS in 1948. Whilst far-reaching
in many respects, this set the scene for a particular configuration of health
and social care services incorporating a tripartite structure[2] of health care
services and a clear boundary between these and the social care services
provided by the local authorities.

The health service reorganization in 1974 incorporated an attempt to
bring together the different sectors; however, as has been pointed out:

---

2 Hospital authorities, executive councils for independent GPs and local health authorities
  responsible for community-based services. Additionally local education authorities
  retained responsibility for school health services.

Although this change was intended to secure a more integrated approach to the provision of health care services, it clearly also had the potential to further deepen the cleavage between health and social care services.

(Hudson 2000: 256)

At the same time the new area health authority boundaries were brought into line with those of the local authorities and new joint consultative committees were created to facilitate the joint development of services (DHSS 1973). These developments coincided with the implementation of the Seebohm Report (1968) which introduced a generic 'social worker' frequently located within a generic team base instead of the previous distinction between child care, mental health and welfare workers located within specific departments.

Within mental health, *Better Services for the Mentally Ill* (DHSS 1975) provided joint funding for new development, but although the trend away from institutional care towards care in the community provided further impetus for joint working between health and social services, progress remained slow and patchy with particular difficulties in transferring resources from the old long-stay institutions to community-based services. There were also concerns expressed about the rising expenditure on residential services. As highlighted in Chapter 3, following a report by the Audit Commission (1986), the government commissioned the Griffiths Report (1988) which led to the White Paper *Caring for People* (DOH 1989) and culminated in the National Health Service and Community Care Act (1990). This Act set the scene for the preparation of joint community care plans and for the implementation of assessment and care management systems.

Over a number of years, shortcomings in different agencies working together were highlighted in several areas, not least those of child protection and mental health. In respect of the former, the inquiry and the subsequent *Report of the Committee of Inquiry into the Care and Supervision Provided in Relation to Maria Colwell* (1974) identified shortfalls in communication and co-ordination between professionals and agencies and led to the setting-up of area review committees to oversee the management of all child abuse cases, involving senior representatives from all the relevant agencies. A number of more recent inquiries culminating in the Victoria Climbie Inquiry (Laming 2003) highlighted continuing difficulties and resulted in the introduction of children's trusts. Unlike care trusts, which are NHS-led, children's trusts are run by local government and emphasis has been placed on a move towards the collaborative integration of children's services, although this remains controversial. In mental health, problems were seen to be related to the 'failure' of community care, as well as to a catalogue of poor inter-agency communication and uncoordinated decisions such as those highlighted by the case of Christopher Clunis (Ritchie 1992). This, together with a number of other similar incidents, led to an increasing emphasis on the need for multi-disciplinary and multi-agency work (DOH 1995).

The 1990s saw a new imperative for working together across the health and social care divide as well as across the old established boundaries. In 1997, the incoming Labour government brought forward its widely publicized agenda for 'joined-up thinking' in tackling a range of health and social problems. The 'modernization' agenda permeated new policy initiatives in relation to health (for example, *The New NHS* [DOH 1997b]; *Modernising Social Services* [DOH 1998a]; *Modernising Mental Health Services* [1998b]) and there has been a renewed emphasis on the sharing of roles and the blurring of boundaries in the interests of providing efficient and cost-effective services.

Further investigation of the continuing debate concerning partnership and joint working, which runs as a constant theme throughout discussion of health and social care policy, reveals a number of tensions and shifts which have implications for the ways in which services are organized and delivered. One aspect of this relates to the continuing historical legacy resulting from the 'competitive imperative' (Hudson and Henwood 2002: 157) embedded within the community care purchaser/provider split. The introduction of market principles into the provision of health and welfare inevitably carried notions of mistrust into the new collaborative environment of joined-up working which, once established, required additional shifts in thinking and 'culture' within organizations to break down the 'Berlin Wall' seen to divide health and social services and referred to by Frank Dobson, Minister of Health, in a speech in 1997 (DOH 1997).

A major thread of this debate, however, concerns the extent to which working together across organizational boundaries, itself facilitated by joint planning, commissioning and funding of services, is an end in itself or a transitional arrangement in the move towards integrated structures. At times this has appeared unclear and the notion of partnership itself has been challenged.

In this context, The Health Act (1999), in addition to facilitating joint financial arrangements between the NHS and local authorities, also created new flexibilities in commissioning and in the integration of services. This was rapidly overtaken by *The NHS Plan* (DOH 2000b), which shifted the agenda from one of partnership to one based on a complete radical redesign of health and social services. Under this Plan, new single multi-purpose legal bodies would commission and be responsible for all local health and social care, and care trusts would commission and deliver primary and community health care as well as social care for older people and other client groups, with social services being delivered under delegated authority from local councils. According to the Plan:

> Care Trusts will usually be established where there is a joint agreement
> at local level that this model offers the best way to deliver better care

services . . . where local health and social care organisations have failed to establish effective joint partnerships – or where services are failing – the government will take powers to establish integrated arrangements through the new Care Trust.

(DOH 2000b: 73)

It is not insignificant that there have been both successes and setbacks amongst the first attempts to establish new joint structures, a number of which have focused on particular aspects of services such as mental health, learning disability and older people. In terms of the casualties, budgetary pressures have been seen to have created tensions and difficulties as well as the need to overcome traditionally diverse ways of working and associated issues of organizational culture, accountability and planning processes. The Buckingham Partnership between the local authority and the local mental health trust, established in 2001, was terminated after three years due to funding difficulties (McCurry 2004) and joint arrangements in Barking and Dagenham have also foundered.

The original intention was that sixteen trusts would be established in April 2002. This figure was later reduced to four and early estimates of eleven care trusts to be established in 2003 were revised to three. The major obstacles have been seen to be financial, legal and employment issues, which have contributed to a wariness and suspicion from all parties (National Primary Care Research and Development Centre [NPCRDC] and the Nuffield Institute 2001). There are also concerns that attempts to emulate the integrated Health and Social Services Boards in Northern Ireland are misplaced as experience suggests that there are similar difficulties there. Hudson and Henwood (2002) point out that the complexities of health and social care require approaches that supersede a concern with organizational structures and hierarchies and are better suited to those that emphasize networks and diverse perspectives including public involvement. It is perhaps not insignificant that the concept of children's trusts is linked to notions of collaboration rather than structural integration and the formation of single integrated organizations.

Notwithstanding the difficulties which have come to be associated with the development of care trusts and partnership, there have been some successes with regard to mental health. One joint trust regarded as successful is the Pennine Care Mental Health NHS Trust which provides specialist mental health services for Bury, Rochdale, Oldham, Tameside and Glossop, serving a total population of nearly 1.2 million. The trust is engaged in working with six primary care trusts and local authorities, voluntary sector organizations and service users and carers to bring about changes in the way that services can be delivered (*The Guardian* 10 March 2004). The intention is to consider various options for change based on the operational needs of the service and its users, founded on system dynamics rather than a managerialist approach. Such an approach highlights cross-discipline solutions and the reality of operational processes, based on clear care pathways rather than being constrained by organizational structures and boundaries.

Bracken and Thomas (2004), as has been seen in Chapter 6, advocate a citizenship approach and draw attention to the 'Sharing Voices' initiative in Bradford. This is funded by Bradford City Primary Care Trust, supported by Bradford District Care Trust, the Community Development Foundation, the Sainsbury Mental Health Centre (SMHC) and the University of Bradford and is located within the Asian Disability Network, a local voluntary sector organization. It is targeted at minority ethnic communities with the aim of developing new thinking and new ways of engaging with these communities. The 'Sharing Voices' initiative prioritizes the development of 'safe spaces' where strategies for coping with stress can be developed and community attitudes towards mental distress can be changed. Support is also offered to those working in places of worship to further enable people in distress to obtain help without the utilization of the language of psychiatry. There are also a variety of self-help initiatives, and befriending schemes and partnerships are being developed with existing statutory and voluntary organizations and businesses to enable people to re-engage in meaningful work.

Within this debate concerning the changing nature and configuration of services, it is important not to overlook the contribution made by the voluntary sector which spans a broad range of large and small organizations. Whilst at a national level, organizations such as MIND and the Mental Health Foundation provide a focus for interest groups, information and political lobbying, at a regional and local level, voluntary sector organizations are frequently key players in the provision of services. In particular, smaller-scale organizations are often recognized for their ability to respond flexibly and creatively to local needs when compared to their statutory counterparts. Additionally, voluntary sector organizations may be seen as being closer to the views of service users and quicker in their ability to move towards models of user-led provision. Not unrelated to this, a further aspect of their provision is the particular contribution which can be made to new ways of working: for example, the development of user-led crisis services or new services involving collaborative relationships between voluntary sector and statutory health and social services.

The voluntary sector is at the forefront of developing alternatives to standard psychiatric services, particularly for women and men from black and minority ethnic communities. The Mental Health Foundation Black Spaces Project (TMHF 2003), for example, highlights the ways in which seven mental health services for minority ethnic communities based in Manchester, Wales, London and the Midlands have evolved to provide specialized services to African-Caribbean and Asian women and men. These projects have included Awaaz, a broad-based service for Asian people in Manchester, the African-Caribbean Community Initiative in Wolverhampton, which runs a day centre and offers support groups as well as sports facilities and IT classes, the Zindaagi project, also in the Midlands, which focuses on supporting young Asian women vulnerable to suicide and self-harm, and the Forward Project in West London, which has concentrated on providing alternatives to psychiatric hospital for African-Caribbean people. The *Black Spaces Report* (Hill 2003b) highlights the importance of working in partnership with key organizations, the need for advocacy to secure black people's rights and the overall necessity of 'empowering users'. Cultural sensitivity to black service users, not dancing to funders' tunes, and the involvement of families and the community in care, have also been seen to be key areas (Hill 2003a, 2003b).

The winner of the 2003 Community Care Awards also draws attention to how the voluntary sector can work in partnership with other agencies to provide responses that are both flexible and innovative. Located within a medicalized frame of reference, yet relying on mutual support, 'No Panic' is a registered charity operated by volunteers whose aim is to 'help the relief and rehabilitation of people who suffer from panic attacks, phobias, obsessive compulsive disorders and other anxiety related disorders' (Community Care Awards 2003: 5). It runs 150 self-facilitating telephone conferencing 'recovery' groups and follow-up befriending groups. An individual can make contact with six other people and proceed with a recovery programme without giving out personal information. The success of the scheme, and the award of the Community Care prize money, have resulted in the recruitment and training of staff from the statutory sector as part of a strategy to shift decision-making into the hands of service users and to promote teleconferencing as a therapeutic tool. Another short-listed finalist promotes equine assisted therapy. Here working with professional therapists and horses offers challenges which in turn facilitate trust, respect, compassionate understanding, communication skills, coping techniques, self-confidence and self-worth. The development of these transferable skills is regarded as effective in enabling those utilizing the scheme to move into full- or part-time work, further education or voluntary work.

One of the difficulties for local organizations has been the need to convince others, including funders and other professional groups, that they are a long way away from the image of amateur volunteers and instead promote a highly professionalized service which can be seen to offer attractive employment conditions and a positive working environment and ethos to those with existing professional qualifications and experience as well as to those without. Notwithstanding this problem more than half a million people are paid employees of the voluntary sector – 569,000 staff or 471,000 full-time equivalents, representing one in 50 of the entire UK paid workforce (National Council for Voluntary Organizations [NCVO] 2004). At a time when public sector employment is decreasing, the voluntary sector has expanded, with social work in the voluntary sector increasing by nearly 69,000 between 1995 and 2000 with at least 40,000 of these being new jobs as opposed to transfers from the statutory sectors (Campbell Robb Society, Guardian.co.uk Thursday 24 January, NCVO 2002).

Further concerns rest on the tension between the ability of voluntary sector organizations to develop and demonstrate innovative work with new projects and approaches alongside the relative financial security of longer-term mainstream service provision. With 37% of the funding for charities coming from the public sector (NCVO 2004), this may leave the sector vulnerable to shifts in public-spending agendas and enmeshed in government priorities. Whilst charities in the UK have assets worth over £70 million, the drive for financial stability may also increase the trend towards service level agreements with statutory providers which in turn leave only limited margins of viability. The consequences of this can be seen in examples of financial crises and the closure of hitherto successful and stable organizations.

With regard to mental health, however, voluntary sector organizations may also be able to step across the boundaries imposed by the distinction between primary care and specialist services and build on a community base to develop wider health partnerships designed to tackle mental health issues as part of a wider holistic approach to public health. The development of the health action zone (HAZ), a means of integrating health services in one area to tackle problems which lead to poor health, and the healthy living centre (HLC), established to promote well-being based on a partnership approach with links to employment and regeneration using lottery funding, can be used as examples. Although the government has moved away from the decentralized flexible approach which characterized the development and operation of HAZs (Fawcett and South 2005), both HAZs and HLCs have offered, and in some cases continue to offer, workable partnerships operating across health and social work/care boundaries which are flexible and particularly amenable to small-scale grass-root voluntary sector organizations.

MENTAL HEALTH AND SOCIAL EXCLUSION

A recognition of wider health matters as well as mental health within this bigger picture inevitably raises the importance of tackling social exclusion, as contained within Standard One of the *National Service Framework for Mental Health* (DOH 1999a). Allied to this is the role of community development in promoting positive mental health and contributing to wider strategies to tackle mental health issues. Underpinning these developments lies a less developed discourse concerning mental health as a more wide-ranging phenomenon which affects everyone and which requires a complex and multi-faceted understanding.

In England, as we have seen, a particular emphasis has been placed on the potential role of a community development approach to improve mental health services for black and minority ethnic communities (National Institute for Mental Health in England [NIMHE] 2003a; Bracken and Thomas 2004).

Alongside a strategy to improve mainstream services in terms of their sensitivity to issues of culture and race, it is proposed that community development workers will both enhance the capacity of black and minority ethnic communities to deal with mental ill-health and contribute to the appropriate development of mainstream services bridging the gap between Western models of care and the practices and values of black and minority ethnic communities. This will be undertaken by considering holistic and culturally appropriate ways of responding to mental health difficulties as well as by identifying and recruiting stakeholders, community leaders and volunteers to engage in local networks and develop self-help projects. Linked to an understanding of models of change within communities, this approach builds on models of community development pioneered in less developed countries and emphasizes the need for community agencies to work together to tackle issues including those of social inclusion and recovery. Whilst this strategy may have much to commend it, its acceptability may, in part, depend on its implementation across all communities, rather than it being confined to black and minority ethnic communities.

As discussed in Chapter 4, the issue of an integrated approach by statutory services to the needs of black and minority ethnic communities is currently underpinned by tensions between a focus on separate services which are seen as necessary to meet needs, and one which emphasizes integration and inclusion within mainstream services which are staffed and resourced to provide a culturally sensitive environment. The issue is summed up by a debate between Bhui and Sashidaran (2003): Bhui sees that greater cultural sensitivity and ownership can only be realized within separate services whilst Sashidaran warns against a 'them and us' situation and against prioritizing difference over inequality and special needs. He goes on to refer to the importance of tackling institutionalized racism and avoiding the bantustanization and colonial discourse of transcultural psychiatry. This approach is echoed in the work of Chantler et al (2001) who, in the context of their work on attempted suicide and self-harm amongst South Asian women, stress the importance of entitlement and citizenship with regard to access to appropriate services.

It is also important to consider the influence of wider societal and economic inequalities on health, recognizing the connection between poor health and indicators of poverty and disadvantage. This again requires a wider agenda for change to bring about health improvements. The *Inside Outside: Improving Mental Health Services for Black and Minority Ethnic Communities in England* (NIMHE 2003) report comments that:

> 'There is a well-established link between structural inequality and variations in health status in all communities'
>
> (2003:10)

Nazroo (1997) suggests that:

'...differences in the rates of mental illness among different ethnic groups might not be a consequence of dimension of ethnicity per se, such as culture or biology, but of the differences in the demographic and socio-economic profiles of different ethnic groups'

(1997: 89)

Such views suggest that the agenda for change must address wider issues of socio-economic disadvantage, inequality and social exclusion (Cameron et al 2003).

As seen in Chapter 4, in relation to social causational arguments, the evidence for the relationship between the higher prevalence of poor mental health and well-accepted markers of inequality and disadvantage comes from a number of sources. The impact of low social position, poor standard of living, limited educational attainment and unemployment on mental health are well recognised, and associated with the impact of gender, highlight that women's mental health is more closely associated with social class status than that of men. Given the preponderance of women who may live in poverty as, for example, single parents, it is also imperative that attempts to address women's mental health are closely allied with strategies to tackle poverty and social exclusion and are not rendered invisible through the use of non-gendered language and explanations (Acheson 1998; Oppenheim and Parker 1996; Hills 1998; Office for National Statistics 2000).

Similarly, to return to the issues of inequality and minority ethnic communities, wide-ranging and joined-up strategies offer the most positive way forward to address the disproportionate incidence of mental health difficulties. Such strategies would recognize the interconnecting and cross-cutting influences of the many factors involved. An appreciation that the main determinants of health are to be found outwith the formal structures of health and social services, also recognizes that it is the upstream factors, namely broad social, economic and environmental conditions, which influence the midstream factors, namely living and working conditions and social and community influences, which in their turn affect the choices and options of individuals and their families.

Overall then it is clear that the notion of community development is beginning to be associated with mental health issues. This can be considered first as part of a wider public health agenda and second as a shift in thinking about mental health from a discourse primarily located in an individualized medical model to one where wider social and environmental aspects are recognized and addressed. Bracken and Thomas (2001) look to 'post-psychiatry' moving beyond its 'modernist' framework to engage with recent government proposals and the growing power of service users. They emphasize the need to look to social and cultural contexts, to place ethics before technology and to work to minimize the medical control of coercive interventions. They see this as positively giving doctors the opportunities to redefine their roles and responsibilities and to engage with community and concepts of citizenship.

This, in turn, leads on to a consideration of notions of social capital.[3] The concept of social capital makes a useful contribution to the understanding of mental health within communities and offers a means of making sense of some of the complex dynamics concerning social inclusion. It highlights the importance of social networks and shared values and trust within communities, supporting the pursuit of shared objectives (McKenzie et al 2002). This may also be viewed as a reciprocal relationship and Sartorius (2003) draws attention to the dynamic between social capital and positive mental health.

This linkage is not entirely unproblematic, however, and requires careful consideration of heterogeneous communities within which there is potential for the continued marginalization and exclusion of minority groups. Again, with regard to black and minority ethnic communities, some mental distress appears to be associated with lower population density within the ethnic group and it is suggested that this may relate to reduced social capital within this group (McKenzie et al 2002).

The challenge to those working in mental health services is the shift required to address the wider upstream factors, already referred to above, rather than those concerned solely with individuals deemed to be in distress or in need of interventions. This will require recognition of the bigger picture at the level of community and locality and the forging of new relationships and associations with those involved in community development, regeneration and renewal.

This links closely with the agenda of the Social Perspectives Network which was created to validate and strengthen the contribution of a social model, already referred to, in further developing understandings and responses to mental health difficulties. The impetus for the Social Perspectives Network originated from a concern that the increasing integration of health and social care would, given the imbalance in terms of resources between the sectors, lead to the reduction of the social model and a corresponding increase in the influence of the medical model. This concern is also fuelled by the changes to the mental health legislation in England and Wales and, as highlighted in Chapter 5, the role of the approved social worker being replaced by that of the approved mental health professional.

An important aspect of the social perspectives agenda includes the need for appropriate user orientated evidence to support social interventions across the spectrum, ranging from the individual to groups and communities. At the individual level this might include work to strengthen family and social networks, gain employment, or access leisure and educational opportunities within the community. For example, the relationship between social

3 A term described by McKenzie et al as 'the forces that shape the quality and quantity of social interactions and social institutions . . . the glue that holds society together' (2002: 280).

functioning, psychological well-being and mental health is well documented, as are the links between the absence of employment and general health problems and premature death. There is also a strong relationship between unemployment and mental health difficulties (Warr 1987; Warner 1994) and it is generally accepted that work that is seen as meaningful to an individual is a major source of self-esteem providing social contact and support, involvement and a sense of personal achievement which overall connects the individual to society.

Evidence suggests that if provided with support, 60% of people with more serious mental health problems can gain and sustain open employment and that success is not linked to diagnosis or severity of symptoms (Secker et al 2001). Additionally, service user views repeatedly stress the importance of social relationships and meaningful activities (Faulkner and Layzell 2000).

Such work is also supported by notions of access associated with the social model of disability and concepts of 'recovery' and social inclusion (Repper and Perkins 2003). Although the emphasis is a little different, this in turn can be linked to the government's strategy for mental health promotion which states that:

> Just as diagnosis is only one part of a person's life, so medical treatment is only one part of the support they need – to cope, to recover and to avoid relapse. The other support – by far the largest part – will come from family, friends, schools, employers, faith communities, neighbourhoods – and from opportunities to enjoy the same range of services and facilities within the community as everyone else.
>
> (DOH 2001d: 59)

Working with mental health at the community level is, for many practitioners, relatively unfamiliar territory. Here it might include working with communities to integrate marginalized groups into mainstream activities, developing self-help networks or creating opportunities for employment and training. Further developing effective working relationships with the voluntary sector and supporting innovative user/survivor-led initiatives are also areas for attention.

However, there are potential risks associated with such a broad and community-based agenda. Not least of these is the possible neglect of some areas as the pendulum swings, as experience has already shown in a number of examples. The development of community-based provision in England and Wales in the 1970s and 1980s, with a similar phenomenon in the USA, albeit within a medical paradigm, led to a proliferation of services available for those experiencing mild to moderate difficulties at the expense of those experiencing longer-term and more serious problems. It has also been suggested that an overriding preoccupation with issues of risk and dangerousness has focused attention on men, leaving women's mental health a neglected area (Payne 1998). A further example, resulting from the amalgamation of health and social care staff within mental health teams, is the increasing gulf between social workers in mental health services and their colleagues working with children and families and the variable development of joint protocols to ensure co-ordination and communication in situations requiring the support of both. In focusing on certain areas, unless great care is taken, by default, attention and consequently resources can be shifted from one area to another. The development of whole systems approaches, by agencies 'providing' mental health services, may serve as a model for wider application across communities and as a means of linking together developments at a number of levels. This might require complex three-dimensional mapping but could contribute to a fundamentally wider understanding, the integration of services across historical divides, and genuine joined-up working. Within such a model, the contribution of the various parties could be recognized and valued. An obvious counter-argument to this approach is the charge that, ultimately, everything is included and that, unless there is a shift in thinking, there is potential for the further medicalization of distress.

A major mechanism which may assist in regulating the impact of change and ensuring that *all* needs are appropriately addressed within a holistic way, recognizing the importance of a social model, may be found if we turn our attention to the public involvement agenda. Issues of user and carer involvement have already been explored elsewhere, but it is important here to locate their influence within the bigger picture. If transformational change is to be effected, fundamental imbalances of power and resources will need to be overturned. Without overlooking the issue of diversity within the user and carer movement, user and carer participation must provide a key driver for change, representing a shift in process as well as in outcome, and requiring a change of seismic proportion in culture and values within mainstream services and organizations if a critical point is to be attained. In the same way that issues of culture within organizations have been seen to resist the efforts by women to transform culture, ethos and working practices (Newman 1995), the shift towards meaningful involvement and participation challenges long-held traditional values which continue to lie beneath the rhetoric of change. As discussed in Chapter 5, the new, if not effectively supported by all stakeholders, will quickly erode to reveal the old. This is borne out by experience elsewhere and summed up by Barnes and Bowl when they refer to 'little detailed evidence of real attitude change among professionals taking place' (2001: 116). It is important to recognize that tension and contradiction are inevitable, but that inclusion and involvement in change processes can result in constructive negotiated outcomes. These outcomes, if not to become inflexible and resistant to change, have to be continually re-negotiated, but this has to be viewed as an integral part of the dynamics of the process. Solutions, by implication, cannot be engineered by imposition and unquestioning adherence to particular orthodoxies, but have to be viewed as temporary and context-specific, highlighting, in turn, those aspects which can be transferred to other situations.

CONCLUDING REMARKS

Inbuilt tension in policy and practice undoubtedly has the capacity to become a negative and destructive force. However, as highlighted, such tension has the potential to be used productively by many groups facing a marked change programme. Tension results in contradiction which in turn provides space for creativity, for innovation and for productively employing key skills, values and knowledge to enable workers to wade through competing directives to work with individuals, groups and communities to build upon and further develop a broad agenda in the field of mental health. What this is, is open to ongoing negotiation both locally and nationally. Existing knowledge bases, skills and values can continue to be subject to critical scrutiny and built upon. Areas regarded as strengths can be prioritized and weaker areas can be re-evaluated and negated or revised. Examples of areas that can be regarded as strengths include: emphasizing the voice, wants and needs of service users, ensuring that micro and macro factors feature in policy and practice, making sure that the importance of co-ordination is highlighted so that both day-to-day and more enduring problem areas can be addressed and ensuring that policy and practice are continually subject to inbuilt, practitioner-orientated 'action' evaluations so that findings continue to inform developments and initiatives.

9   Conclusion

'As an experience, madness is terrific . . . and in its lava I still find most of the things I write about.' Virginia Woolf, who committed suicide in 1941
(Nicholson and Trautmann 1976)

This book has taken as its starting point the understanding that mental health and mental ill-health are contested, multi-faceted and changing concepts. The key tenets of psychiatry and psychiatric systems have changed over time, as have the perspectives of those who see themselves or who are seen by others as experiencing various forms of mental distress. At particular points different views have been promoted and presented as 'the' way both to conceptualize and to respond to mental distress. It has been contended in this book that the ways in which positions and understandings become fixed have to be subject to ongoing critical interrogation, with full account being taken of the reasons for the formation of allegiances around particular positions by a variety of interest groupings.

It is useful at this point to revisit the key arguments which have been presented in this book. The three broad overlapping themes highlighted in Chapter 2 relate to first, the importance of not adopting a fixed position in relation to mental distress; second, the utility of having a range of flexible frameworks so that individual difficulties can be located within explanatory frames that are regarded as helpful and supportive and which enable an individual to position himself or herself as well as to critically interrogate the way in which she or he has been positioned; and third, the pervasive attraction of illness models which have dividing practices embedded within them, yet which can also be used as a point of challenge. These themes have informed the ways in which theoretical perspectives and policy and practice frameworks have been explored. Similarly, the importance of placing users/survivors centre stage has been emphasized throughout. In this context it has been maintained that those with experience of mental distress have as valid a contribution to make as any other. It has also been contended that it is necessary to recognize that here, as in psychiatry, positions can become impervious to change. It could be argued that given the imbalance of power between psychiatrists and users/survivors that has prevailed since psychiatry emerged as a science, giving prominence and predominance to the traditionally devalued position is a constructive step. Smart (1992) and Flax (1992), however, have pointed out that if prevailing knowledge claims are going to be interrogated then this has to apply to all knowledge claims including those of users/survivors. Flax (1992) draws attention to the dangers of 'innocent knowledge', where some knowledge claims can be regarded as being untainted by power relations. She also highlights how such knowledge claims can result in certain areas becoming uncritically defended with particular perspectives being adopted unquestioningly.

The concept of 'innocent knowledge' can be considered in relation to the social model of disability. With regard to disabled people, this model has proved to be an impressive vehicle for bringing about change. However, in order to succeed, issues of diversity and experiences of impairment have been subsumed and have given way to political arguments. Wilson and Beresford (2002) regard the social model of disability as providing opportunities for users/survivors to come together to exert greater pressure for user/survivor-directed change. However, they are aware of both positive and negative aspects encapsulated within this specifically targeted and politically orientated model. They also raise the issue of the distinction between 'impairment' and disability and express concern that the residual association between 'impairment' and biological characteristics of the body and mind can easily result in 'mental illness' being seen as a form of physical/sensory impairment. A further 'reification' of mental illness would, they argue, be unhelpful for users/survivors, although they suggest that there is considerable scope for exploring the socially constructed nature of 'impairment' (Wilson and Beresford 2002: 155).

When reviewing an area which is as contested as mental distress, the importance of historical context cannot be underestimated. In Chapter 3 the enduring features of the policy and practice framework have been seen to include an ongoing concern with risk and dangerousness and the perceived need for containment and coercive responses. The arguments presented challenge the view that risk can be measured and predicted and, drawing from Langan (1999), focus on how values and social, political, economic and cultural factors affect definitions and assessments of risk. Attention has also been drawn to how prevailing political, social and economic trends influence mental health policy and practice and the reform of the Mental Health Act (1983) has been cited as an example of this. However, it is also pertinent that, despite reflecting dominant political, social and economic drivers, this legislation has lacked consensus support from a significant number of diverse yet involved stakeholders.

Taking an historical perspective also draws attention to the influence of modernist ways of thinking. Belief in science, progress and rationality still underpins Western psychiatric perspectives and informs the view that it is possible to objectify and systematically and clinically to study dysfunction in isolation from social and cultural factors. This has resulted in aspects related to difference and diversity not being sufficiently acknowledged or regarded as contributing factors in the social causation or social construction of mental ill-health.[1] The setting of 'scientific' research approaches against those that are more qualitatively orientated has led to reflexive, ontological, ethical and epistemological underpinnings (that is, how we view the world, why we view it in this way and how we utilize 'knowledge'), not being seen as particularly relevant for scientific enquiry and not being critically interrogated. It has been argued in Chapter 4 that differences associated with gender and ethnicity do not operate in isolation, but intersect and interact with other differences such as social class and sexuality. Accordingly, the importance of avoiding compartmentalization has been highlighted and, particularly in relation to Asian women and black African-Caribbean women, the need to recognize multi-faceted and interconnected features has been emphasized. It has been noted that the ways in which difference has been responded to have been many and varied, but it is obvious that, despite some innovative developments, pertinent issues are a long way from being resolved.

In relation to mental distress, attention has been drawn throughout this book to how positions often become polarized, adversarial and defensive. Bracken and Thomas (2001) have looked at the ways in which psychiatry has been subject to ongoing attack and criticism resulting in defensive reactions to challenge and change. They pertinently state:

> . . . although patients complain about waiting lists, professional attitudes, and poor communication, few would question the enterprise of medicine itself. By contrast, psychiatry has always been thus challenged. Indeed, the concept of mental illness has been described as a myth. It is hard to imagine the emergence of 'antipaediatrics' or 'critical anaesthetics' movements . . .
>
> (Bracken and Thomas 2001: 724)

As discussed in Chapters 6 and 8, Bracken and Thomas want to move beyond the modernist confines of psychiatry and by means of 'post-psychiatry' to ensure that social, political and cultural realities become central to understandings about mental health. Their assertion that empirical knowledge has a limited utility and that a simple cause-and-effect model is inadequate to take account of the interconnectedness between events, reactions and social networks and the complexities of values and assumptions, contests simplistic polarizations between psychiatrists and users/survivors. The ways in which they challenge the view that psychiatric theory is neutral,

---

1 'Ill-health' has been used instead of 'mental distress' at this point to emphasize the point being made.

objective and disinterested, thereby weakening the case for medical control of coercive assessment and treatment models, can also be seen as dynamic in that it removes a rigid and constraining element and constructively facilitates negotiation between users/survivors, psychiatrists, policy makers, family members and practitioners.

The importance of carer and user/survivor involvement (with the different requirements of each being fully acknowledged) in all aspects of existing provision, including planning and service delivery, has been highlighted in Chapter 7. Whilst there are pitfalls, it has been recognized that new ways of working together, which challenge traditional dichotomies between 'providers' and 'receivers', need to be developed to counter existing barriers.

With regard to current policy, prevailing tension, paradox and inconsistency have been highlighted as a means both of facilitating a constructive critique and as a way of emphasizing how these aspects can be productive. It has been argued that these unintended features can create space to manoeuvre to bring about challenge and change, and to contest inflexible and procedurally orientated transitions from policy into practice. 'Seamlessness' has been seen as a concept more amenable to the rhetoric of policy directives rather than to practice and as generally more aspirational than actual. It has been pointed out that an emphasis on seamlessness can result in papering over the cracks rather than engagement in a process which opens these up for more detailed inspection. It has been contended that it is the latter which, although more time-consuming and complex, can result in longer-lasting and, if an inclusive approach to change is adopted, more viable outcomes.

The importance of the voluntary sector and the effective utility of voluntary/statutory collaborations have been particularly emphasized in Chapter 8, although the problems associated with small-scale, voluntary endeavours have been noted. As indicated, many projects, particularly those focusing on community involvement, emerged as a result of health action zone funding. These were influenced by previous community participation initiatives, but the funding was not extended as originally envisaged and subsequent programmes (and Sure Start serves as a good example) found themselves having to comply with a more than comprehensive set of centrally driven performance targets. This had led to friction between the push of community involvement and the pull of centralized performance measures. It has been noted that a focus on community involvement, social inclusion, and the utilization of social capital is somewhat at odds with an emphasis on centrally driven perfomance management and budgetary targets. If community involvement in arenas such as mental health is to move forward, there are significant areas which need to be addressed. These include commitment by all stakeholders, clarification about the level and extent of participation, transparency in terms of how targets and goals are decided upon, the making of decisions about how progress towards the agreed goals is to be monitored, agreement about what constitutes representation, and the commitment of resources such as time, expertise and support as well as money over guaranteed time periods. However, it has also been recognized that community involvement will not solve issues of discrimination and the alienation of those regarded as 'other'. Indeed if key issues relating to discrimination are not directly tackled and continually reinforced, then, as noted in Chapter 8, community involvement could result in further alienation and in the renewed dominance of medical understandings and responses. However, currently there can be seen to be a dynamic relationship between social capital and positive mental health and this is an area which clearly warrants further constructive exploration.

CONCLUDING REMARKS

Finally it is important to emphasize that a central focus of this book has been the exploration of the dynamic and rapidly changing kaleidoscope of concepts and ideas concerning mental health which underpin current debates. Not dissimilar to the children's toy that rotates pieces of coloured glass to form ever-changing patterns, the pieces of this kaleidoscope form various configurations, with each highlighting a plethora of different aspects and themes. The significant difference, however, is that, rather than valuing each permutation of the pieces equally with their unique shapes and colours, the importance of context is emphasized. Accordingly, in particular contexts competing claims can be fully acknowledged, different understandings and concomitant implications can be appreciated and power imbalances can be recognized. Like a revolving kaleidoscope, the different configurations warrant action in terms of dynamic and flexible theory, policy and practice arrangements.

Bibliography

Acheson D (1998) Independent inquiry into inequalities in health report. London: HMSO

Ackerman L (1997) Development, transition or transformation: the question of change in organizations. In Van Eynde D, Hoy J and Van Eynde D, eds, *Organization Development Classics*. San Francisco: Jossey Bass

Alaszewski A (1998) Risk in modern society. In Alaszewski A, Harrison L and Manthorpe J, eds, *Risk Health and Welfare*. Buckingham: Open University Press

Allott P and Loganathan L (2002) *Discovering Hope for Recovery from a British Perspective*. Birmingham: Centre for Community Mental Health, University of Central England

American Psychiatric Association (1980) *Diagnostic and Statistical Manual of Mental Disorders*, 3rd edition (DSM-III). Washington, DC: American Psychiatric Association

American Psychiatric Association (1994) *Diagnostic and Statistical Manual of Mental Disorders*, 4th edition (DSM-IV). Washington, DC: American Psychiatric Association

Arksey H (2002) *Services to Support Carers of People with Mental Health Problems: A Briefing Paper*. London: National Co-ordinating Centre for NHS Service Delivery and Organisation Research and Development

Armstrong D (1995) The rise of surveillance medicine. *Sociology of Health and Illness* 17, 3: 393–404

Arshad J and Johal B (1999) Culture club. *Nursing Times* 95, 9: 66–67

Atkinson R (1999) Discourses of partnership and empowerment in contemporary British urban regeneration. *Urban Studies* 36, 1: 59–72

Audit Commission (1986) *Making a Reality of Community Care*. London: Audit Commission

Audit Commission (2001) *Change Here! Managing Change to Improve Local Services*. London: Audit Commission

Bagley C (1971) Mental illness in immigrant minorities in London. *Journal of Biosocial Science* 3: 449–459

Baistow K (1994) Liberation or regulation? Some paradoxes of empowerment. *Critical Social Policy* Spring 1994/5 Winter 14(3): 34–46

Barnes M (1997) *Care Communities and Citizens.* London: Longman

Barnes M and Bowl R (2001) *Taking Over the Asylum – Empowerment and Mental Health.* Basingstoke: Palgrave

Barnes M and Maple N (1992) *Women and Mental Health: Challenging the Stereotypes.* Birmingham: Venture Press

Barnes M, Bowl R and Fisher M (1990) *Sectioned: Social Services and the 1983 Mental Health Act.* London: Routledge

Bartlett A, King M and Phillips P (2001) Straight talking: an investigation of the attitudes and practice of psychoanalysts and psychotherapists in relation to gays and lesbians. *British Journal of Psychiatry* 179: 545–549

Bean P, Bingley W, Bynoe I (1991) *Out of Harm's Way.* London: MIND

Beck U (1992) *Risk Society: Towards a New Modernity,* trans M Rutter. London: Sage Publications

Beresford P (2000) Service users' knowledges and social work theory: conflict or collaboration. *British Journal of Social Work* 30, 4: 489–503

Beresford P (2002a) Turning the tables. *Openmind,* July/August, 116: 16–17

Beresford P (2002b) Participation and social policy: transformation, liberation or regulation? In Sykes R, Bochel C and Ellison N, eds, *Social Policy Review 14: Developments and Debates: 2001–2002.* Bristol: The Policy Press

Beresford P (2003a) On the way to work. *Community Care Magazine* 19–25 June: 20

Beresford P (2003b) *A new approach to service user involvement in research and development,* presentation to the National User Network conference. Shaping Our Lives (25 June)

Beresford P and Croft S (1993) *Citizen Involvement: A Practical Guide for Change.* Basingstoke: BASW/Macmillan

Berzins K (2003) *Legislation Affecting Carers of People with Mental Health Problems.* European Federation of Associations of Families of Mentally Ill People. www.eufami.org [accessed 24 June 2004]

Bhugra D and Jones P (2001) Migration and mental health. *Advances in Psychiatric Treatments* 3: 216–223

Bhugra D and Mastrogianni A (2004) Globalization and mental disorder. *British Journal of Psychiatry* 184: 10–20

Bhugra D, Baldwin D S, Desai M and Jacob K S (2000) Attempted suicide in West London 11. *Intergroup Comparisons: Psychological Medicine* 29, 5: 1131–1139

Bhui K and Sachidaran S (2003) Should there be separate services for ethnic minority groups? *British Journal of Psychiatry* 182: 10–12

Boyd W D (1994) *Preliminary Report on Homicide.* The Steering Committee of the Confidential Inquiry into Homicides and Suicides by Mentally Ill People. London: Department of Health

Bracken P and Thomas P (2001) Post-psychiatry: a new direction for mental health. *British Medical Journal* 322: 724–727

Bracken P and Thomas P (2004) Out of the clinic and into the community. *OpenMind* March/April, **126**: 13

Bracken P, Greenslade L, Griffin B and Smyth M (1998) Mental health and ethnicity: an Irish dimension. *British Journal of Psychiatry* **172**: 103–105

Bremner J and Hillin A (1993) *Sexuality, Young People and Care*. London: CCETSW

Bridget J and Lucille S (1996) Lesbian Youth Support Information Service (LYSIS): developing a distance support agency for young lesbians. *Journal of Applied Social Psychology* **6, 5**: 355–364

British Psychological Society (2000) *Recent advances in understanding mental illness and psychotic experiences*. London: British Psychological Society. www.bps.org.uk/publications

Brodrib S (1992) *Nothing Matters: A Feminist Critique of Postmodernism*. Melbourne: Spinnifex

Brooker C, James A and Redhead E (2003) *National Continuous Quality Improvement Tool for Mental Health Education*. Durham: Northern Centre for Mental Health

Broverman D, Clarkson F, Rosencratz P et al (1970) Sex role stereotypes and clinical judgements of mental health. *Journal of Consulting and Clinical Psychology* **34**: 1–7

Browne D (1997) *Black People and Sectioning: The Black Experience of Detention under the Civil Sections of the Mental Health Act*. Little Rock Publishing

Brown G W and Harris T O (1978) *The Social Origins of Depression*. London: Tavistock

Brown GW, Harris TO and Hepworth C (1995) Loss and Depression: a patient and non-patient comparison. *Psychological Medicine* **25**: 7–21

Burns T, Knapp M, Catty J, Healey J, Henderson J, Watt H and Wright C (2001) Home treatment for mental health problems: a systematic review. *Health Technology Assessment:* 5–15

Burr V (1995) *An Introduction to Social Constructionism*. London: Routledge

Bury M (1998) Postmodernity and health. In Scrambler G and Higgs P, eds, *Modernity Medicine and Health: Medical Sociology Towards 2000*. London: Routledge

Busfield J (1996) *Men, Women and Madness: Understanding Gender and Mental Disorder*. Basingstoke: Macmillan

Busfield J, ed (2001) Rethinking the sociology of mental health. In *Sociology of Health and Illness*. Oxford: Blackwell

Cameron M, Edmans T, Greatley A and Morris D (2003) *Community Renewal and Mental Health: Strengthening the Links*. London: King's Fund and National Institute of Mental Health in England (NIMHE)

Campbell P (1996) The history of the user movement in the United Kingdom. In Heller T, Reynolds J, Gomm R, Muston R and Pattison S, eds, *Mental Health Matters – A Reader*. London: Macmillan/Open University

Carling P J and Allott P (1999) *Beyond Mental Health Services: Integrating Resources and Support in the Local Community.* Birmingham: NHS Executive

Carpenter L and Brockington I F (1980) A study of mental illness in Asians, West Indians and Africans in Manchester. *British Journal of Psychiatry* **137**: 201–205

Carr S (2004) *Has Service User Participation made a Difference to Social Care Services?* Bristol/London: The Policy Press/Social Care Institute for Excellence

Carrier J and Kendall I (1995) Professionalism and interprofessionalism in health and community care: some theoretical issues. In Owens P, Carrier J and Horder J, eds, *Interprofessional Issues in Community and Primary Health Care.* London: Macmillan

Centre for Policy on Ageing (1998) *Defining Difference* Occasional Paper No 1, London: CPA

Chantler K, Burman E, Batsleer J and Bashir C (2001) *Attempted Suicide and Self-Harm (South Asian Women).* Manchester: Metropolitan University, Women's Studies Research Centre

Charcot J M (1887–8) Charcot the clinician: the Tuesday lessons, excerpts from *Nine Case Presentations on General Neurology*, ed and trans C G Goetz. Delivered at the Sapetrière Hospital in 1887–1888. New York: Raven Press, in Porter R, ed (1991) *The Faber Book of Madness.* London: Faber & Faber

Clare A (1988) *Psychiatry in Dissent: Controversial Issues in Thought and Practice,* 3rd edn, London: Tavistock Publications

Chesler P (1972) *Women and Madness.* New York: Doubleday

Cochrane R (1977) Mental illness in immigrants to England and Wales. *Social Psychiatry* **12**: 25–35

Cochrane R (1983) *The Social Creation of Mental Illness.* London: Longman

College of Occupational Therapists and Royal College of Psychiatrists (2002) *Mental Health and Occupation in Participation.* A consensus statement. www.cot.org.uk

Community Care Awards (2003) *Community Care Magazine,* 27 November–3 December: 40–41

Cooper B (2003), Evidence-based mental health policy: a critical appraisal. *British Journal of Psychiatry* **183**: 105–113

Cope R (1989) The compulsory detention of Afro-Caribbeans under the Mental Health Act. *New Community* **15**, 3: 343–356

Coppock V and Hopton J (2000) *Critical Perspectives on Mental Health.* London: Routledge

Corker M and French S, eds (1999) *Disability Discourses.* Buckingham: Open University Press

Corti L and Dex S (1995) Information carers and employment. *Employment Gazette* **103**: 101–107

Craik C, Auston A, Chacksfeild L, Richards G and Schell D (1998) College of Occupational Therapists: position paper on the way ahead for research and practice in mental health. *British Journal of Occupational Therapy* **61, 9**: 290–302

Croft S and Beresford P (1992) *From Paternalism to Participation: Involving People in Social Services*. Open Services Project, York: Joseph Rowntree Foundation

Crossley N (2000) Emotions, psychiatry and social order: a Habermasian approach. In Williams S, Gabe J and Calnanm M, eds, *Health, Medicine and Society: Key Theories, Future Agendas*. London: Routledge

Davies N, Lingham R and Simms A (1995) *Report of the Inquiry into the Circumstances Leading to the Death of Jonathan Newby (A Volunteer Worker) on 9th October 1993 in Oxford*. Oxford: Oxfordshire Health Authority

Dean G, Walsh D, Downing H and Shelly P (1981) First admissions of native-born and immigrants to psychiatric hospitals in south-east England 1976. *British Journal of Psychiatry* **139**: 506–512

Department of Health (1989) *Caring for People: Community Care in the Next Decade and Beyond*, Cm 849. London: HMSO

Department of Health (1995) *Building Bridges: A Guide to the Arrangements for Inter-Agency Working for the Care and Protection of Severely Mentally Ill People. The Health of the Nation*. London: HMSO

Department of Health (1997a) *Speech by the Minister of Health*, Frank Dobson, 21 October, ref. 97: 290

Department of Health (1997b) *The New NHS: Modern, Dependable*. London: The Stationery Office

Department of Health (1998a) *Modernising Social Services*. London: HMSO

Department of Health (1998b) *Modernising Mental Health Services: Safe, Sound and Supportive*. London: The Stationery Office

Department of Health (1999a) *National Service Framework for Mental Health: Modern Standards and Service Models*. London: The Stationery Office

Department of Health (1999b) *Effective Co-ordination in Mental Health Services: Modernizing the Care Programme Approach – a Policy Booklet*. London: The Stationery Office

Department of Health (2000a) *A Health Service of All the Talents*. London: The Stationery Office

Department of Health (2000b) *The NHS Plan: A Plan for Investment, a Plan for Reform*. Cm. 4818-1. London: The Stationery Office

Department of Health (2000c) Mental Health National Service Framework Workforce Planning Education and Training Underpinning Programme: Interim Report by the Workforce Action Team. London: www.doh.gov/pdfs/nsfmentinterim.pdf

Department of Health (2000d) *Reforming the Mental Health Act*. Cm5016 London: Department of Health

Department of Health (2001a) *Health and Social Care Act Section 11.* London: The Stationery Office

Department of Health (2001b) *Journey to Recovery.* London: The Stationery Office

Department of Health (2001c) *Reforming the Mental Health Act – Part One: the New Legal Framework.* London: The Stationery Office, www.doh.gov.uk/menhlth

Department of Health (2001d) *Making it Happen- A Guide to Mental Health Promotion.* London: The Stationery Office

Department of Health (2002a) *Women's Mental Health: Into the Mainstream: Strategic Development of Mental Health Care for Women.* London: The Stationery Office

Department of Health (2002b) *Requirement for Social Work Training.* London: The Stationery Office

Department of Health (2002) *Developing Services for Carers and Families of People with Mental Illness.* London: Department of Health

Department of Health (2003a) *Delivering Race Equality: A Framework for Action.* London: The Stationery Office

Department of Health (2003b) *Mental Health Policy Implementation Guide: Support, Time and Recovery (STR) Workers.* London: The Stationery Office

Department of Health (2003c) *Inside/Outside: Improving Mental Health Services for Black and Minority Ethnic Communities in England.* London: National Institute for Mental Health in England

Department of Health (2005) Hospital Episode Statistics by Primary Diagnosis. http://www.dh.gov.uk/PublicationsAndStatistics/Statistics/HospitalEpiso deStatistics/HESFreeData/HESFreeDataList/fs/en?CONTENT_ID=4097 375andchk=HLM%2BM4 Accessed 12.4.05.

Department of Health and Social Security (1971) *Hospital Services for the Mentally Ill.* London: HMSO

Department of Health and Social Security (1973) *A Report from the Working Party on Collaboration between the NHS and Local Government on Its Activities to the End of 1972.* London: HMSO

Department of Health and Social Security (1975) *Better Services for the Mentally Ill.* London: HMSO

Department of Health and Social Security (1977) *The Role of Psychologists in the Health Service (the Trethowen Report).* London: HMSO

Derrida J (1978) *Writing and Difference* (trans Bass P). Chicago: University of Chicago Press

Disability Discrimination Act (1995). London: The Stationery Office

Di Stefano C (1990) Dilemmas of difference. In Nicholson L J, ed, *Feminism/ Postmodernism.* London: Routledge

Dixon L B and Lehman A F (1995) Family interventions for schizophrenia. *Schizophrenia Bulletin* 21: 631–643

DOH See Department of Health

Dohrenwend B and Dohrenwend B S (1977) Sex differences in mental illness: a reply to Gove and Tudor. *American Journal of Sociology* **82**: 1336–1341

Dominelli L (2002) *Anti-oppressive Social Work Theory and Practice*. New York: Palgrave/Macmillan

Double D (2002a) The limits of psychiatry. *British Medical Journal* **324**: 900–904

Double D (2002b) *Redressing the biochemical imbalance*. [http://www.critpsynet.freeuk.com/doublesep.htm]

Douglas M and Wildavsky A (1982) *Risk and Culture*. London: University of California Press

Dover S and McWilliam C (1992) Physical illness associated with depression in the elderly in community based and hospital patients. *Psychiatric Bulletin* **16**: 612–613

Dowson S (1990) *Keeping it Safe: Self Advocacy by People with Learning Difficulties and the Professional Response*. London: Values into Action

Duggan M, Cooper A and Foster J (2002) *Modernising the Social Model in Mental Health: A Discussion Paper*. London: Social Perspectives Network for Modern Mental Health, TOPSS (www.topss.org.uk/uk_eng)

Ehrenreich B and English D (1979) *For Her Own Good: 150 Years of the Experts' Advice to Women*. London: Pluto Press

Eichenbaum L and Orbach S (1983) *What do Women Want?* London: Michael Joseph

Elvin E (2003) Name change may end paternalism. *Community Care Magazine*, 18–24 September: 22

Escher S, Romme M and Buiks A (1998) Small talk – voice hearing in children. *Openmind*, July/August, **92**: 12–13

Excell J and Mayes D (2003) Who needs a day centre? *OpenMind*, March/April, **120**: 26

Fallon P (1999) *The Report of the Committee of Inquiry into the Personality Disorder Unit, Ashworth Special Hospital*. Cm. 4194–ii. London: The Stationery Office

Fanon F (1967) *Black Skin, White Masks*. London: MacGibbons Kee

Faulkner A H and Cranston K (1998) Correlates of same-sex sexual behaviour in a random sample of Massachusetts high school students. *American Journal of Public Health* **88**, 2: 262–266

Faulkner A and Layzell S (2000) *Strategies for Living: A Report of User Led Research into People's Strategies for Living with Mental Distress*. London: The Mental Health Foundation

Faulkner A and Thomas P (2002) User-led research and evidence-based medicine. *British Journal of Psychiatry* **180**: 1–3

Fawcett B (2000) *Feminist Perspectives on Disability*. Harlow: Prentice-Hall

Fawcett B and Featherstone B (1996) 'Carers' and 'caring': new thoughts on old questions. In Humphries B, ed, *Critical Perspectives on Empowerment*. Birmingham: Venture Press

Fawcett B and Hearn J (2004) Researching others: epistemology, experience standpoints and participation. *Social Science Research Methodology 7*, 3: 201–218

Fawcett B and South J (2005) Community involvement and primary care trusts: the case for social entrepreneurship. *Critical Public Health* in press

Fawcett B, Featherstone B and Goddard J (2004) *Contemporary Child Care Policy and Practice*. Basingstoke: Palgrave/Macmillan

Fernando S (1991) *Mental Health, Race and Culture*. Basingstoke: Macmillan/ MIND

Fernando S (1995) *Mental Health in a Multi-Ethnic Society*. London: Routledge

Fernando S (2002) *Cultural Diversity, Mental Health and Psychiatry: The Struggle Against Racism*. London: Routledge

Fernando S (2003) Inside/Outside. *Openmind*, July/August, **122**: 22–23

Fernando S, Ndegwa D and Wilson M (1998) *Forensic Psychiatry, 'Race' and Culture*. London: Routledge

Finch J and Groves D (1983) *Labour of Love: Women, Work and Caring*. London: Routledge & Kegan Paul

Finkelstein V (1991) Disability: an administrative challenge? In Oliver M, ed, *Social Work: Disabled People and Disabling Environments*. London: Jessica Kingsley

Fishbach RL and Herbert B (1997) Domestic violence and mental health: correlates and conundrums across and within cultures. *Social Science and Medicine 25*: 7–21

Fisher M (1997) Man-made care: community care and older male carers. *British Journal of Social Work* **24**: 659–680

Flax J (1992) The end of innocence. In Butler J and Scott J, eds, *Feminists Theorise the Political*. London: Routledge

Fook J (2002) *Social Work: Critical Theory and Practice*. London: Sage Publications

Fossey E, Happell B, Harvey C et al (2001) Research in mental disorders and mental health practice. In McDermott F, Meadows G, Singh B, Wadsworth Y, eds, *Mental Health in Australia: Collaborative Community Practice*. Oxford: Oxford University Press

Foucault M (1965) *Madness and Civilization*. New York: Random House

Foucault M (1981) Question of method: an interview with Michael Foucault. *Ideology and Consciousness* 8: 1–14

Fox N (2000) The ethics and politics of caring: postmodern reflections. In Williams S, Gabe J and Calnanm M, eds, *Health, Medicine and Society: Key Theories, Future Agendas*. London: Routledge

Francis E (1988) Black people, dangerousness and psychiatric compulsion. In Brachx A and Grimshaw C, eds, *Mental Health Care in Crisis*. London: Pluto

Francis E (2003) A light in a dark room. *Community Care Magazine* 23–29 October: 30–32

Fraser N and Nicholson L (1993) Social criticism without philosophy: an encounter between feminism and postmodernism. In Docherty M, ed, *Postmodernism: A Reader*. Hemel Hemstead: Harvester Wheatsheaf

Frost N (2002) Evaluating practice. In Adams A, Dominelli L and Payne M, *Critical Practice in Social Work*. Basingstoke: Palgrave

General Social Care Council (2002) *Accreditation of Universities to grant Degrees in Social Work*. London: GSCC

Giddens A (1998) *The Third Way: The Renewal of Social Democracy*. Cambridge: Polity Press

Glover-Thomas N (2002) *Reconstructing Mental Health Law and Policy*. London: Butterworth

Goffman E (1961) *Asylums*. Harmondsworth: Penguin

Goldberg D and Huxley P (1980) *Mental Illness in the Community: The Pathways to Psychiatric Care*. London: Tavistock

Goldberg D and Huxley P (1992) *Common Mental Disorders, a Bio-Social Model*. London: Tavistock/Routledge

Goldie N (2003) Vulnerable to cuts. *Community Care Magazine* 13–19 February: 36–37

Golding J (1997) *Without Prejudice: Lesbian, Gay and Bisexual Mental Health Awareness Research*. London: MIND

Goodwin R E and Mitchell D, eds (2000) *The Foundation of the Welfare State, Volume 1*. Cheltenham: Edward Elgar

Gorman J (1992) *Out of the Shadows*. Policy paper. London: MIND

Goss S and Miller C (1995) *From Margin to Mainstream: Developing User and Carer Centred Community Care*. York: Joseph Rowntree Foundation

Green M, Karban K, Nazar N, Shah R, South J and Tilford S (2002) *South Asian Women: Mental Health Needs and Services in South Leeds*. Leeds: Leeds Metropolitan University

Griffiths R (1988) *Community Care: Agenda for Action*. London: HMSO

Grobe J, ed (1995) *Beyond Bedlam: Contemporary Women Psychiatric Survivors Speak Out*. Chicago: Third Side Press

Harding S (1993) Rethinking standpoint epistemology: what is strong objectivity? In Alcoff L and Potter E, eds, *Feminist Epistemologies*. London and New York: Routledge, pp 67–99

Harrison G, Owens D and Holton A (1984) Psychiatric hospital admissions in Bristol 11: social and clinical aspects of compulsory admission. *British Journal of Psychiatry* 145: 605–611

Harrison G et al (1989) *Psychological Medicine* 19: 683–696

Harrison M (2002) Perils of engagement. *Mental Health Today* September: 28–30

Heise L L, Pitinguy J and Germain A (1994) *Violence Against Women: The Hidden Health Burden*. World Bank Discussion Paper no. 1255

Hepworth D (2000) *Black and Minority Ethnic Carers and Access to Carer's Assessment.* York: University of York, Social Policy Research Unit

Hicks N (1997) Evidence-based health care. *Bandolier* 4(4): 49

Hill N (2003a) Safe passage. *Community Care Magazine* 30 October–5 November: 36–37

Hill N (2003b) *Black Spaces Report.* London: The Mental Health Foundation

Hills J (1998) *Income and Wealth: the latest evidence.* York: Joseph Rowntree Foundation

Hirschman (1998) Service users as consumer. In Hugman R, ed, *Social Welfare and Social Value – The Role of Caring Professions.* London: Macmillan

HMSO (1992) *Big Black and Dangerous: Report of the Committee of Inquiry into the Death in Broadmoor Hospital of Orville Blackwood and a Review of the Death of Two Other Afro-Caribbean Patients.* London: HMSO

Hogman G and De Vleesschanwer R (1996) *The Silent Partners – An Overview of the EUFAMI Survey into Carers' Needs.* European Federation of Associations of Families of Mentally Ill People. www.eufami.org [accessed 24 June 2004]

Horwitz A V (2002) *Creating Mental Illness.* Chicago: Chicago University Press

Howe G (1995) *Working with Schizophrenia: A Needs Based Approach.* London and Bristol: Jessica Kingsley

Huang M C and Slevin E (1999) The experiences of carers who live with someone who has schizophrenia: a review of the literature. *Mental Health and Learning Disabilities Care* 3, 3: 89–93

Hudson B (2000) Inter-agency collaboration – a sceptical view. In Brechin A, Brown H and Eby M, eds, *Critical Practice in Health and Social Care.* London: Sage Publications

Hudson B and Henwood M (2002) The NHS and social care: the final countdown? *Policy & Politics* 30, 2: 153–166

Huxley P and Thornicroft G (2004) Social inclusion, social quality and mental illness. *British Journal of Psychiatry* 182, 4: 289–290

Improvement and Development Agency (1999) Summary of Information collected by EO/IdeA on the mental health workforce

Independent Inquiry into the Death of David Bennett (2003) Cambridge: Norfolk, Suffolk and Cambridgeshire Strategic Health Authority

Ineichen B (1990) The mental health of Asians in Britain. *British Medical Journal* 300: 1669–1670

Ineichen B, Harrison G and Morgan GH (1984) Psychiatric hospital admissions in Bristol: 1. Geographical and ethnic factors. *British Journal of Psychiatry* 145: 600–604

Ingleby D, ed (2004) *Critical Psychiatry – the Politics of Mental Health*, 2nd edn, London: Free Association Books

Inquiry into the Death of David Bennett (2003) Cambridge: Norfolk Suffolk and Cambridgeshire Strategic Health Authority. http://guardian.co.uk/sys-files/society/documents/2003/02/12/Bennett.pdf

Jackson S (1992) The amazing deconstructing woman. *Trouble and Strife* 25: 25–31

Johnstone L (2000) *Users and Abusers of Psychiatry*, 2nd edn, London: Routledge

Jones K (1972) *A History of the Mental Health Services*. London: Routledge & Kegan Paul

Kaplan H and Sadock B (1995) *Comprehensive Text Book of Psychiatry*, Vols 1 and 2, 6th edn, Baltimore: Williams and Wilkins

Kawachi I, Kennedy BP and Glass R (1999) Social capital and self-rated health: a contextual analysis. *American Journal of Public Health* 89: 1187–1193

King M and McKeown E (2003) *The Mental Health and Social Wellbeing of Gay Men, Lesbians and Bisexuals in England and Wales*. London: MIND

Kirmayer L J (2001) Cultural variations in the clinical presentation of depression and anxiety: implications for diagnosis and treatment. *Journal of Clinical Psychiatry* 62 (suppl. 13): 22–28

Laing R (1965) *The Divided Self*. Harmondsworth: Penguin

Laming H (2003) *The Victoria Climbie Inquiry: Report of an Inquiry by Lord Laming*. Cm. 5730. Norwich: The Stationery Office

Langan J (1999) Assessing risk in mental health. In Parsloe P, ed, *Risk Assessment in Social Care and Social Work*. London: Jessica Kingsley

Leason K (2003) Mental health 'tsar' admits services suffer from institutional racism. *Community Care Magazine* 17–23 July: 18–19

Leff J P and Vaughan C (1981) The role of maintenance therapy and relatives' expressed emotion in relapse in schizophrenia: a two year follow up. *British Journal of Psychiatry* 139: 102–104

Lewis G, Gewirtz S and Clarke J (2000) Expanding the social policy imaginary. In Lewis G, Gewirtz S and Clarke J, eds, *Rethinking Social Policy*. London: Sage/Open University

Light D W and Cohen A (2003) *Commissioning Mental Health Services: Experiences from the United States of America*. London: Sainsbury Centre for Mental Health

Linford Rees W L, Lipsedge M and Ball C, eds (1996) *A Textbook of Psychiatry*. London: Hodder

Lister R (1997) *Citizenship: Feminist Perspectives*. Basingstoke: Macmillan

Lister R (2002) *Citizenship: Feminist Perspectives*, 2nd edn, Basingstoke: Palgrave

Littlewood R (1992) Psychiatric Diagnosis and Racial Bias: Empirical and Interpretive Approaches. *Social Science and Medicine* 34(2): 141–149

Littlewood R and Cross S (1980) Ethnic minorities and psychiatric services. *Sociology of Health and Illness* 2: 194–201

Littlewood R and Lipsedge M (1981) Acute psychotic reactions in Caribbean-born patients. *Psychological Medicine* 11: 289–335

Lloyd K and Moodley P (1992) Psychotropic Medicine and Ethnicity: an inpatient survey. *Social Psychiatry and Social Epidemiology* 27(2): 95–101

McCurry P (2004) Under pressure. *Care and Health* 18 February 55: 28–29

MacFarlane L (1998) *Diagnosis: Homophobic.* London: Project for Advice Counselling and Education (PACE)

McGovern D and Cope R (1987) The compulsory detention of males of different ethnic groups with special reference to offender patients. *British Journal of Psychiatry* 150: 505–512

Mckenzie K, Whitley R and Weich S (2002) Social capital and mental health. *British Journal of Psychiatry* 181: 280–283

MacPherson Report (1999) *The Stephen Lawrence Inquiry: Report of an Inquiry by Sir William MacPherson of Cluny.* London: The Stationery Office

Marriott D (2000) *On Black Men.* Edinburgh University Press

Martin J (1984) *Hospitals in Trouble.* Oxford: Blackwell

Maudsley H (1887) Body and mind: an inquiry into their connection and mutual influence specially in reference to mental disease. Referred to in Porter R, ed (1991) *The Faber Book of Madness.* London and Boston: Faber

Maynard M (1994) 'Race' gender and the concept of 'difference in feminist thought. In Afshar H and Maynard M, eds, *The Dynamics of 'Race' and Gender, Some Feminist Interventions.* London: Taylor & Francis

Meadows G and Sing L B, eds (2002) *Mental Health in Australia: Collaborative Community Practice.* Oxford: Oxford University Press

Mental Health Act Commission *Eighth Biennial Report* 2002. London: HMSO

Midwinter E (1994) *The Development of Social Welfare in Britain.* Buckingham: Open University Press

Monbiot G (2001) *Captive State: The Corporate Take Over of Britain.* London: Pan

Moore M, Beazley S and Maelzer J (1998) *Researching Disability.* Buckingham: Open University Press

Morgan S and Juriansz D (2002) Practice-based evidence. *OpenMind,* March/April, 114: 12–13

Morrall P (1997) Professionalism and community psychiatric nursing: a case study of four mental health teams. *Journal of Advanced Nursing* 25: 1133–1137

Morris J (1993) *Pride Against Prejudice.* London: Women's Press

Mulvaney J (2000) Disability, impairment or illness? The relevance of the social model of disability to the study of disability. *Sociology of Health & Illness* 5: 582–601

Murphy E (1991) *After the Asylums: Community Care for People with Mental Illness.* London: Faber & Faber

Murray JL and Lopez AD (1996) *The global burden of disease: A comprehensive assessment of mortality and disability from diseases, injuries and risk factors in 1990 and projected to 2020.* Boston: Harvard School of Public Health, World Health Organization

National Confidential Inquiry into Suicide and Homicide by People with Mental Illness (2001) *Safety First: Five Year Report of the National Confidential Inquiry into Suicide and Homicide by People with Mental Illness* London: Department of Health

National Council for Voluntary Organizations (2004) *The United Kingdom Voluntary Sector Almanac.* London: National Council for Voluntary Organizations.

National Institute for Clinical Excellence (2002) *Schizophrenia: Core Interventions in the Treatment and Management of Schizophrenia in Primary and Secondary Care.* London: NICE

National Institute for Mental Health in England (2003a) *Cases for Change: Emerging Areas of Service Provision.* London: Department of Health

National Institute for Mental Health in England (2003b) *Cases for Change: A Review of the Foundations of Mental Health Policy and Practice 1997–2002.* London: Department of Health

National Institute for Mental Health in England and Sainsbury Centre for Mental Health Joint Workforce Support Unit (2004) *The Ten Essential Shared Capabilities – A Framework for the Whole of the Mental Health Workforce.* Draft (June)

National Working Group on New Roles for Psychiatrists (2004) *New Roles for Psychiatrists.* London: British Medical Association

Nazroo J (1997) *Ethnicity and Mental Health.* London: Policy Studies Institute

Nettleton S and Gustafsson U (eds) (2002) *The Sociology of Health and Illness Reader.* Cambridge: Polity Press

New Burr V (1995) *An Introduction to Social Constructionism.* London: Routledge

Newham Inner City Multifund and Newham Asian Women's Project (1998) *Young Asian Women and Self-Harm.* London: Newham Asian Women's Project

Newman J (1995) Gender and cultural change. In Itzin C and Newman J, (eds), *Gender Culture and Organizational Change.* London: Routledge

Nicholson N and Trautmann, eds *The Letters of Virginia Woolf,* Vol 2. New York: Harcourt/Brace 1975–80

Nolan P (1993) *A History of Mental Health Nursing.* London: Chapman & Hall

Norfolk, Suffolk and Cambridgeshire Strategic Health Authority (2003) *Inquiry into the Death of David Bennett.* Cambridge: Norfolk, Suffolk and Cambridge Strategic Health Authority

Nuffield Foundation (1997) *User Perspectives on Research.* Leeds: Community Care Division. Nuffield Foundation

Oakley A (1981) *Subject Women*. London: Martin Robertson

Office for National Statistics (2002) *The Mental Health of Carers*. London: The Stationery Office

Office for National Statistics (2000) *Psychiatric Morbidity Among Adults Living in Private Households*. London: HMSO

Office of the Deputy Prime Minister (2003) *Mental Health and Social Exclusion Consultation Document*. London: Social Exclusion Unit

Oliver M (1996) *Understanding Disability: From Theory to Practice*. London: Macmillan

Ong YL (2001) Psychiatric services for black and minority ethnic elders. Council report CR103. London: Royal College of Psychiatrists www.rcpsych.ac.uk/publications

Onyett S (2003) *Teamworking in Mental Health*. Basingstoke: Palgrave/Macmillan

Onyett S, Heppleston T and Bushnell D (1994) A national survey of community mental health team structure and process. *Journal of Mental Health* 3: 145–194

Oppenheim C and Harker L (1996) *Poverty: the facts*. London: Child Poverty Action Group

Parker I, Georgaca E, Harper D, McLaughin T and Stowell-Smith M (1995) *Deconstructing Psychopathology*. London: Sage

Parton N (1998) Risk, advanced liberalism and child welfare: the need to rediscover uncertainty and ambiguity. *British Journal of Social Work* 28, 1: 5–27

Patterson C H (1986) *Theories of Counselling and Psychotherapy*, 4th edn, New York: Harper & Row

Payne S (1998) Hit and miss – the success and failure of psychiatric services for women. In Doyal L, ed, *Women and Health Services – An Agenda for Change*. Buckingham: Open University Press

Peplau H (1952) *Interpersonal Relations in Nursing*. New York: G P Putman

Pereira C (1997) Introduction. In Bornat J, Johnson J, Pereira C, Pilgrim D and Williams F, eds, *Community Care: A Reader*, 2nd edn, Basingstoke: Open University Press/Macmillan

Perkins R (2003a) Day Centre Debate. *OpenMind* 120: 26

Perkins R (2003b) *OpenMind*, May/June, 121: 6

Perkins R (2004) The Guilds. *OpenMind* 128:14

Perkins R and Repper J (1998) *Dilemmas in Community Mental Health Practice: Choice or Control*. Oxford: Radcliffe Medical Press

Perkins R and Repper J (1999) *Working Alongside People with Long-Term Mental Health Problems*. Cheltenham: Stanley Thorne

Persaud R (1993–4) Comment. *OpenMind*, Vol 24, December–January

Pierson C (1998) *Beyond the Welfare State*, 2nd edn, Cambridge: Polity Press

Pilgrim D and Rogers A (1994) *A Sociology of Mental Health and Illness*. Buckingham: Open University Press

Pilgrim D and Rogers A (1999) *A Sociology of Mental Health and Illness*, 2nd edn, Buckingham: Open University Press

Pilgrim R (1998) Divided mind. *OpenMind*, July/August, **92**: 23

Porter R (1991) (ed) *The Faber Book of Madness*. London: Faber & Faber

Power S (2001) Joined-up thinking? Inter-agency partnerships in education action zones. In Riddell S and Tett L, eds, *Education, Social Justice and Inter-Agency Working*. London and New York: Routledge, pp 14–28

Prior L (1993) *The Social Organization of Mental Illness*. London: Sage Publications

Prior P M (1999) *Gender and Mental Health*. Basingstoke: Macmillan

Project for Advice Counselling and Education (1998) *Diagnosis Homophobic*. London: PACE

Ramon S (1996) *Mental Health in Europe: Ends, Beginnings and Rediscoveries*. Basingstoke: Macmillan

Redfern M (2001) *The Report of the Royal Liverpool Children's Inquiry*. London: The Stationery Office

Report of the Committee of Inquiry into the Care and Supervision Provided in Relation to Maria Colwell (1974) London: HMSO

Report of the Royal Commission on Lunacy and Mental Disorder (Cmd. 2700) (1926) London: HMSO. Available at http://www.bopcris.ac.uk/bopall/ ref8569.html

Repper D and Brooker C (2002) *Avoiding the Washout*. Durham: Northern Centre for Mental Health

Repper J and Perkins R (1998) Assessing the needs of people who are disabled by serious ongoing mental health problems. In Baldwin S, ed, *Needs Assessment and Community Care: Clinical Practice and Policy Making*. Oxford: Butterworth-Heinemann

Repper J and Perkins R (2003) *Social Inclusion and Recovery*. London: Baillière Tindall

ReSistors (2002) *Women Speak Out: Women's Experiences of using Mental Health Services in Leeds and Proposals for Change*. Leeds: ReSisters, Leeds Women and Mental Health Action Group

Rethink (2003) *Under Pressure – the Impact of Caring on People supporting Family Members or Friends with Mental Health Problems*. Kingston upon Thames: Rethink

Rethink (2004) *Carers Support*. www.rethink.org/services.carers_support.html #CESP [accessed 9 July 2004]

Ritchie J (1994) *The Report of the Inquiry into the Care and Treatment of Christopher Clunis*. London: HMSO

Rivers I (1995) Mental health issues among young lesbians and gay men bullied in school. *Health and Social Care in the Community* **3**: 380–383

Roberts K and Harris J (2002) *Disabled People in Refugee and Asylum Seeking Communities*. Joseph Rowntree Foundation Findings. York: Joseph Rowntree Foundation (www.jrf.org.uk)

Rochefort D and Goering P (1998) More a link than a division: how

Canada has learned from US. *Mental Health Policy Health Affairs* **17**, 5: 110–127

Rogers A and Pilgrim D (1996) *Mental Health Policy in Britain: A Critical Introduction*. Basingstoke: Macmillan

Rogers A and Pilgrim D (2003) *Mental Health and Inequality*. Basingstoke: Palgrave

Romme M and Escher S (1993) *Accepting Voices*. London: MIND

Rose D, ed (2001) *Users' Voices: The Perspectives of Mental Health Service Users on Community and Hospital Care*. London: Sainsbury Centre for Mental Health

Rose D (2003) User involvement in research, different truths and critics. In *Different Truths: User Control and Involvement in Mental Health Research and Evaluation*. The Mental Health Foundation Virtual Conference, December. www.connects.org.uk/conferences/default.asp?codeItemID=26 [accessed 18 June 2004]

Rose D, Fleischmann P, Tonkiss F, Campbell P and Wykes T (2003) *Review of the Literature: User and Carer Involvement in a Mental Health Context*. Report to NHS Service Delivery and Organization Research and Development Programme

Rose H and Bruce E (1995) Mutual care but differential esteem: caring between older couples. In Arber S and Ginn J, eds, *Connecting Gender and Ageing: A Sociological Approach*. Buckingham: Open University Press, pp 114–128

Royal Commission on Lunacy and Mental Disorder Report (1926) London: HMSO

Sainsbury Centre for Mental Health (1997a) *More Than Just A Friend – the Role of Support Workers in Community Mental Health Settings*. London: SCMH

Sainsbury Centre for Mental Health (1997b) *Pulling Together: The Future Roles and Training of Mental Health Staff*. London: SCMH

Sainsbury Centre for Mental Health (2000) *The Capable Practitioner*. London: SCMH

Sainsbury Centre for Mental Health (2002) *Breaking the Circles of Fear: A Review of the Relationship between Mental Health Services and African and Caribbean Communities*. London: SCMH.

Sainsbury Centre for Mental Health (2003) *The Mental Health Service User Movement in England*. Policy Paper 2. London: SCMH

Salize H J and Dressing H (2004) Epidemiology of involuntary placement of mentally ill people across the European Union. *British Psychiatry* **184**: 163–168

Sartorius N (2003) Social capital and mental health. *Current Opinion in Psychiatry* **16**, supplement 2: S101–S105

Sashidharan S P (1993) Afro Caribbeans and schizophrenia: the ethnic vulnerability hypothesis re-examined. *International Review of Psychiatry* **5**: 129–144

Sashidharan S (2003) Comments in 'Author of mental health report says government diluted racism findings. *Community Care Magazine* 17–23 July

Sayce L (2000) *From Psychiatric Patient to Citizen (Overcoming Discrimination and Social Exclusion)*. Basingstoke: Macmillan

Scheff T (1966) *Being Mentally Ill: A Sociological Theory*. Chicago: Aldine

Scull A (1977) *Decarceration: Community Treatment and the Deviant – a Radical View*. Englewood Cliffs, NJ: Prentice Hall

Secker J, Grove B and Seebohm P (2001) Challenging barriers to employment, training and education for mental health service users. *Journal of Mental Health* 10: 395–404

Seebohm F (Chair) (1968) *Report of the Committee on Local Authority and Allied Social Services*. Cmnd. 3703. London: HMSO

Seed P (1973) *The Expansion of Social Work in Britain*. London: Routledge & Kegan Paul

Seligman M (1975) *Helplessness*. San Francisco: Freeman

Shah A (1998) The psychiatric needs of ethnic minority elders in the UK. *Age and Ageing.* May 1998

Shaikh S (1985) Cross-cultural comparison, psychiatric admissions of Asian and indigenous patients in Leicestershire. *International Journal of Social Psychiatry* 31: 3–11

Shakespeare T (2000) The social relations of care. In Lewis G, Gewirtz S and Clarke J, eds, *Rethinking Social Policy*, London: Sage Publications

Shaw A and Shaw I (2001) Risk research in a risk society. *Research Policy and Planning* 19, 1:1–22

Shifrin T (2004) Diving for charity pearls. *Guardian Society* Wednesday 18 February

Showalter E (1987) *The Female Malady: Women, Madness and English Culture 1830–1980*. London: Virago Press

Skultans V (1979) *English Madness: Ideas on Insanity, 1580–1890*. London: Routledge & Kegan Paul

Simoni-Wastila L (2000) The use of abusable prescription drugs: the role of gender. *Journal of Women's Health and Gender Based Medicine* 9: 289–297

Smart B (1993) *Postmodernity*. London: Routledge

Smart C (1992) Feminist approaches to criminology or postmodern woman meets atavistic man. In Gelsthorpe L and Morris A, eds, *Feminist Perspectives in Criminology*. Milton Keynes: Open University Press

Smith J (2002) *Death Disguised: The First Report of the Shipman Inquiry*. London: HMSO

Stacey M (1988) *The Sociology of Health and Healing*. London: Unwin Hyman Ltd

Steering Committee of the Confidential Inquiry into Homicides and Suicides by Mentally Ill People (1994) *A Preliminary Report on Homicide*. London: Department of Health

Stein L and Test M (1980) Alternative mental hospital treatment: 1. Conceptual model: treatment program and clinical evaluation. *General Psychiatry* **37**: 392–397

Szasz T S (1971) *The Manufacture of Madness*. London: Routledge & Kegan Paul

Tansella M and Burti L (2003) Integrating evaluative research and community-based mental health care in Verona, Italy. *British Journal of Psychiatry* **183**: 167–169

Taylor B (2004) Men, masculinity and mental health. Unpublished PhD thesis. University of Bradford

Taylor D, ed (1996) *Critical Social Policy: A Reader*. London: Sage Publications

Taylor P and Gunn J (1984) Violence and psychosis: risk of violence among psychotic men. *British Medical Journal* **288**: 1945–1949

Taylor P and Gunn J (1999) Homicides by people with mental illness: myth and reality. *British Journal of Psychiatry* **174**: 9–14

The Mental Health Foundation (1997) *Knowing Our Own Minds: A Survey of how People in Emotional Distress Yake Control of their Own Lives*. London: The Mental Health Foundation

The Mental Health Foundation (2001) *Turned Upside Down: Developing Community-based Crisis Services for 16–25 Year Olds Experiencing a Mental Health Crisis*. London: The Mental Health Foundation

Timms N (1964) *Psychiatric Social Work in Great Britain (1939–1962)*. London: Routledge & Kegan Paul

Titmuss R (1963) *Essays on the Welfare State*. London: Allen & Unwin

Treacher A and Baruch G (1980) Towards a critical history of the psychiatric profession. In Ingleby D, ed *Critical Psychiatry: The Politics of Mental Health*. Harmondsworth: Penguin

Trethowen Report, see Department of Health and Social Security (1977)

Tudor K (1996) *Mental Health Promotion – Paradigms and Practice*. London: Routledge

Users' Voices (2001) *The Perspectives of Mental Health Service Users on Community and Hospital Care*, ed Rose D. London: Sainsbury Centre for Mental Health

Ussher J (1991) *Women's Madness: Misogyny or Mental Illness?* Hemel Hempstead: Harvester Wheatsheaf

Wallcraft J and Bryant M (2003) *The Mental Health Service User Movement in England*. London: Sainsbury Centre for Mental Health

Warner R (1994) Recovery from schizophrenia. In *Psychiatry and Political Economy*, 2nd edn, London: Routledge

Warr P (1987) *Unemployment and Mental Health*. Oxford: Oxford University Press

Weinberg A and Huxley P (2000) An evaluation of the impact of voluntary sector family support workers on the quality of life of carers of schizophrenia sufferers. *Journal of Mental Health* **9**, 5: 495–503

Wessley S, Castle D, Der G and Murray R (1991) Schizophrenia and Afro-Caribbeans: a case-control study. *British Journal of Psychiatry* **159**: 795–801

Wheeler E (1994) Doing black mental health research. In Afshar H and Maynard M, eds, *The Dynamics of 'Race' and Gender: Some Feminist Interventions*. London: Taylor & Francis

Williams F (1992) Somewhere over the rainbow: universality and diversity in social policy. In Manning N and Page R, eds, *Social Policy Review 4*. London: Social Policy Association

Williams F (1994) Michele Barrett: from Marxist to poststructuralist feminism. In George V and Page R, eds, *Modern Thinkers on Welfare*. Hemel Hempstead/ London: Harvester Wheatsheaf

Williams F (1996) Postmodernism feminism and the question of difference. In Parton N, ed, *Social Theory, Social Change and Social Work*. London: Routledge

Williams F (2001) In and beyond New Labour: towards a new political ethics of care. *Critical Social Policy* **21**, 4: 467–493

Wilson A and Beresford P (2002) Madness, distress and postmodernity: putting the record straight. In Corker M and Shakespeare T, eds, *Disability/Postmodernism: Embodying Disability Theory*. London: Continuum

Wilton T (1998) Gender, sexuality and health care: improving services. In Doyal L, ed, *Women and Health Services – An Agenda for Change*. Buckingham: Open University Press

World Health Organization (1990) *International Statistical Classification of Diseases and Related Health Problems,* 10th revision (ICD-10). Geneva: WHO

World Health Organization (2000) *Women's Mental Health: An Evidence Based Review*. Geneva: World Health Organisation

Younghusband E L (1964) *Social Work and Social Change*. London: George Allen & Unwin

Index

Printed and bound by CPI Group (UK) Ltd, Croydon, CR0 4YY

01/11/2024

01782636-0009